101

Agility Drills

Patrick McHenry, MA, CSCS*D, PES
Joel Raether, Med, CSCS

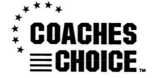

COACHES ☰ CHOICE™

ISBN: 978-1-58518-902-1
Library of Congress Control Number: 2004107138
Cover design: Brennan Tiffany
Book layout: Studio J Art & Design
Front cover photo: Brennan Tiffany

Coaches Choice
P.O. Box 1828
Monterey, CA 93942
www.coacheschoice.com

Dedication

To my family, especially Michele and Morgan, for all their support.

—Patrick McHenry

I would like to dedicate this book to my mother and father,
who have guided me in all facets of my life to get me where I am today.

—Joel Raether

Acknowledgments

This book is a compilation of experience gained from many years of talking with coaches, attending coaching clinics, and working with athletes. It would be impossible to thank everyone who has helped me over the years, but I would like to give a special thanks to all the coaches, especially Randy Huff, Jamie Woodruff, and the rest of the staff and students at Ponderosa High School who use these drills day in and day out. I would also like to give thanks to the National Strength and Conditioning Association for all their help and support over the years.

—Patrick McHenry

I would like to thank Mike Sanders and Drew Bodette (University of Denver) for helping me develop this approach to agility training. I would also like to thank Jon Larsen (University of Nebraska at Kearney) for his support and teachings in this field. Lastly, I would like to thank my co-author, Patrick McHenry, for allowing me to help with this project.

—Joel Raether

Preface

Many coaches still feel that agility is a quality you are born with and cannot be enhanced. Research has shown that this belief is not true and agility can be improved upon if worked on correctly. The question is: "What is correct?"

We do not proclaim to have all the answers or drills. In this book, we are simply showing you what has worked for us and other colleagues over the past years. You must take these drills and make them your own. Each athlete and situation is different, so adjust your program to meet your athletes' needs. Do not think that one drill will fit every situation or that all athletes will progress in the same manner.

This book was designed so you can take any drill, whether it is level I, II, or III, put it into your practice, and it will enhance your athletes' skills. As a coach, know the drill and the desired outcome so you can correct any flaws that may occur.

At the end of the book, we have included both the references and recommended reading. The list offers a wide variety of resources where you can find answers to just about any questions you may have about agility training.

In closing, it is not the drill that makes athletes great; it is athletes' hard work and dedication to performing the skill that is elicited from the drill that will make them great.

Contents

1

Introduction to Agility Training

In today's world of competitive sports, the emphasis on training for sports has become paramount. In this realm, the emergence of agility drills as a means to increase sports performance has come to the forefront. In the "Essentials of Strength Training and Conditioning," the term *agility* is referred to as the ability to stop, start, and change the direction of the body or body parts rapidly and in a controlled manner (3). Moreover, agility is a trainable (51, 4, 49) skill that needs to be worked on continuously, demands proper mechanics in the upper and lower body, and has specific guidelines that need to be followed so training does not just become another form of conditioning (50, 34).

Numerous variables can be trained to aid in the body's ability to move. In sports, an athlete must be able to start and stop as quickly as possible in any direction. In many cases, these movements are repetitious in fashion and numerous in footwork complexities. Therefore, the faster an athlete can accelerate and decelerate repeatedly, the higher the likelihood of success. Moreover, the enhanced ability to control the body may lower injury implications. The use of agility training can increase an athlete's ability to accelerate, decelerate, and control the body through limitless movement patterns. If an athlete can increase movement pattern efficiency and also decrease time to execute given courses, the probability of increased sports performance would also seem warranted.

The goal of this book is to provide a multitude of agility drills, which vary in complexity while using numerous implements that can be used to increase such factors as footwork, acceleration, deceleration, and body control. Moreover, this book will demonstrate a systematic approach to introducing agility drills to any level of athlete and will show how to progress athletes from basic agility drills to more complex drills as skill acquisition increases.

Getting Started

Before any training session begins, it is essential to perform a proper warm-up. The warm-up should resemble the movements that are to be performed. The warm-up prepares the muscles and joints by increasing blood flow, intermuscular temperature, and intramuscular coordination, as well as increasing joint viscosity via synovial fluids (52). Contrary to popular belief, the warm-up routine should not include static stretching. Static stretching needs to be performed, but should be done post-exercise. The rationale behind static stretching is that it is a relaxation tool for the musculature and joints. Muscle spindles and Golgi tendon organs (GTO) are receptors in the muscle that are sensitive to length and tension. These receptors are activated when a muscle is stretched or tension is increased. When these receptors are initiated, they act to protect the muscle from injury by inhibiting or "guarding" the muscle from stretching further or adding additional tension. When a static stretch is held, these receptors allow the muscle to stretch beyond normal resting parameters. Research supports the notion that if static stretching is performed prior to exercise bouts, these receptors may allow the muscle to stretch beyond normal limits, thus increasing injury possibilities. This lowered response from the receptors may be attributed to static stretching, which lowers the muscle receptors' responsiveness and/or sensitivity. Prior to performing ballistic type movements (i.e. running, jumping), initiating a relaxed state in the muscles and joints may not only be harmful, but may be detrimental to performance in the strength and power athlete. In fact, research indicates that static stretching can produce a 5 to 30 percent acute decrement in strength and power production (3).

The warm-up routine should resemble the types of movements that will be performed during the practice or event. The movements performed in agility drills and most athletic endeavors are dynamic in nature, therefore the warm-up routine should consist of drills that are dynamic as well. Such drills include high knees, carioca, skips, shuffles, etc. By performing these dynamic drills, the muscles and receptors are prepared for movements that may be encountered during exercise bouts.

The following is an example of a dynamic warm-up routine. Note that this routine is merely an example of drills that will ready your athletes. Any combination of drills can be performed that may be more sport-specific for the dynamic warm-up. The warm-up should last approximately 15 to 30 minutes to properly warm the muscles and joints. The athletes should have reached the point of sweating by the end of the dynamic warm-up.

Sample Dynamic Warm-up Routine

- Jog 100 meters
- Skip 100 meters
- Walking lunges 10 meters
- Side lunges 10 meters
- Butt kicks 10 meters
- High knees 10 meters
- Ankle hops 10 meters

- "A" skips 10 meters
- "B" skips 10 meters
- Carioca 10 meters
- Shuffles 10 meters
- Toy soldiers 10 meters
- Power skips 20 meters
- Accelerations 30-60 meters

Equipment Needs

Nearly all agility drills can be performed with very minimal equipment. The implements that will be needed for drills in this book include cones, 12-inch hurdles, four- to six-inch boxes, and speed ladders. If you do not have access to these implements, you can easily substitute other items. Common substitutes for cones include t-shirts, shoes, and hats. Aerobic steps can be used for boxes and athletic tape is an easy way to create speed ladders. Hurdles may be the hardest to find an alternative for, but can be substituted for, as long as safety is considered. Hurdles need to be easily moveable in regards to athletes hitting them while going over them. If the hurdle is too high or unmovable, the risk of injury may be high if the athlete contacts the hurdle while performing a drill.

A good rule of thumb for substituting an agility course implement is to make sure that safety is the first and foremost concern. If an object is going to be used, make sure that if an athlete contacts, knocks over, or steps on the object, injury possibilities are minimal.

Body Positioning

Before performing agility drills, it is essential to gain an understanding of basic body positioning and the mechanics that are necessary to improve agility performance. Having the upper body and lower body working together is essential to the performance of the athlete. For instance, sprint times can be affected by as much as 10 percent if proper arm mechanics are not used (7). It is important to point out that straight-ahead (SA) speed is not the same as agility speed. In fact, researchers (53) had one group of athletes work on SA speed and another on agility and found that both groups improved, but only in the skill that was practiced and not in the other. Thus, it is crucial to understand that agility skills must be improved through agility training.

The most basic mechanical function that an athlete should learn is the positioning of the hips during any direction change. To make the most effective and fluent transition from moving in one direction to another direction, the hips must be lowered (Figure 1-1). The lowering of the hips is paramount in agility training. This positioning allows the athlete to decelerate quickly and also puts the athlete in position to move in any direction immediately. Notice in Figure 1-1 that the upper body is over the hips and the feet are in position to drive in any direction from this point.

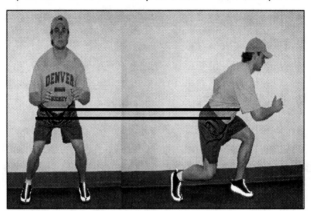

Figure 1-1

Another coaching method for acceleration and deceleration is to understand shin angles during both acceleration and deceleration. Shin angles can be most easily seen in a positive, negative, or neutral angle. The angle of the shin is marked by the angle formed from the bottom of the foot to the lower leg where the ankle joint is the fulcrum. During acceleration, the angle of the shin should be positive (Figure 1-2) or in a driving position to move the body forward. Likewise, during deceleration, the angle of the shin should resemble a negative angle. Any time that the angle of the shin is positive, the body is in an accelerating position. When the shin is at a negative angle, the body is in a decelerating or braking mode. The more pronounced the angle, the more quickly the athlete will accelerate or decelerate.

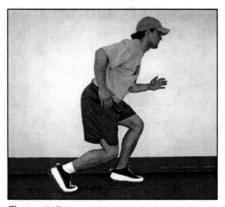

Figure 1-2

Any time that a direction change is made, the athlete must lower the hips to help prepare the body to decelerate. The upper body must lead this process as well. If the hips lower and the upper body leans too far forward, the athlete will have to take many additional steps to stop because of the momentum of the upper body. As the hips lower, the upper body should remain over the hips or slightly leaned back so that the lower body can control deceleration.

If the athlete can learn to lower the hips and manage upper body control, the legs will be put into a drive position every time, which will allow the athlete to change directions more quickly and more effectively. This point of balance is referred to as the body's center of mass (19). This balance point can be located at 55 percent of height in women and 57 percent of height in men. This center of balance may be the most essential component of agility training.

An athlete's sense of balance or what is referred to as a "kinesthetic awareness" (49) will determine the athlete's ability to perform agility movements. Therefore, it is crucial to start athletes in agility-like training at early ages. Sport scientists have shown that children who perform agility-like drills during the prepubescent stages of development demonstrate a higher degree of motor control patterns later in life (45,37). This finding does not necessarily mean that an older athlete who has not previously performed agility drills cannot receive benefits from agility training; it merely means that the more basic motor patterns an athlete can master at an early age, the easier it will be to become proficient at sport-specific techniques later on (34).

Designing Agility Programs

The designing of agility programs has not been widely discussed or examined, while the concept of periodization with regards to weight training has been conceptualized for years. Just as with other forms of training, agility training must have a form of progression and planning in order for advancement and skill acquisition to have maximal benefits (49). The methodology that has been established by the authors of this book is derived from similar concepts of traditional periodization models. This system includes teaching of basic footwork, moving from one-dimensional drills to multi-variant drills, and generally progressing from drills more simple in fashion to the highest complexities. As training status increases, so does the complexity level of footwork components in the drills, as well as the number of footwork components. The progression of drill selection will also develop from closed courses to open courses, which will be discussed later in the readings.

The object of periodizing agility drills is to ensure that athletes can gain footwork proficiency while progressively increasing complexity. This goal is accomplished by classifying drills according to levels of complexity. For example, drills that are only one-dimensional, such as a forward run into a backpedal, would be a level I drill because only one footwork component is being performed. When the athlete shows competence with one-dimensional drills, a new level of drills should be introduced. Level II drills should incorporate more direction changes and more footwork variables than level I drills do. One example of a level II drill is performing a forward run into a backpedal while moving laterally. As the athlete's performance increases and level II drills are mastered, the athlete should advance to more complex, level III drills.

In level III, drills will include increased footwork components and also increased directional components. The athlete will have to perform numerous direction changes as well as numerous footwork variables in the same drill. An example of a level III drill would be a T-test where the athlete would have to perform running, shuffling, and backpedaling while moving forward, backward, and laterally.

It is imperative to note that the athletic level of your athlete will determine how quickly the progression through levels will occur. Coaches need to know where their athletes are athletically. They also need to keep in mind where the athletes are in training (in-season, pre-season, or off-season). The drills are set up in a manner to teach proper motor patterns. Teaching basic drills and progressing to more complex drills will "teach proper sequencing of motor unit firing" (49).

It is also important to note that when proficiency of drills is apparent it does not mean that the drill should never be performed again. It is essential to periodically perform lower-level drills to maintain sound footwork mechanics. Also, when specific times of the year allow (i.e. off-season, pre-season), it may be beneficial to start progressions over and fine-tune footwork and body mechanics before advancing to higher levels of drills. Athletes that are injured or coming off of rehabilitation can also use the progression of drills to aid in the return to full playing status.

Coaches need to keep in mind that agility training is not conditioning. If you are truly focusing on the development of the athlete's agility, then you must build rest times into training sessions (49, 48, 34, 4, 19). Coaches should also alternate training intensity—scheduling heavy, medium, and light days—so that the athlete can maximize recovery between workouts. Agility training utilizes the neuromuscular system and the ATP-PC system (41, 43, 36), which means that recovery is imperative between agility sets to ensure maximal effort by the athlete. If drills exceed 10 seconds in length per repetition, different energy systems will be used that will initiate more of a conditioning effect such as speed endurance, which may not be the goal of training. Excessive drill duration will lead to fatigue and technique breakdown, which may cause poor motor habits and poor overall drill quality.

As the athlete progresses with drills, it is essential to keep drills moving in a direction of sport-specificity. For instance, during the off-season, it would not be as important for the athlete to be performing very specific drills (45). As the training moves from the off-season to the pre-season, the drills should shift toward more sport-specific drills (47). The more specific the training drills can be to the sport, the more effective they will be in enhancing competitive performances (40, 5, 19, 9). The coach should also make athletes aware of the purpose of drills and the progression plan. Research has shown that if the athlete does not recognize transfer of learning, then it may be detrimental to the athlete's performance (27). When you show them the importance of the skill being performed in the drill, the athletes become aware of the "elements that need to be transferred" (9).

Closing Remarks

All of the drills that are displayed in this book are designed to help athletes reach higher levels of performance. By following the guidelines that have been established in this book, coaches can implement quality agility programs into their programs. Keep in mind that quality of drills should be the goal. Make sure that your athletes use good technique and give maximum effort during each training session, because it is not the course itself that will enhance performance but how the course is being performed.

The progressions in this book have been established as a way for coaches to have a systematic approach to implementing agility programs. Using these progressions, nearly all combinations of footwork components can be worked on. Make sure that your athletes show proficiency with all drills before progressing to higher-level drills. This guideline may be the most crucial aspect of the system. If athletes are progressed too fast, sound footwork and overall technique will not reach desired levels.

Coaches should keep in mind that agility drills are endless and only limited to your imagination. All of the drills displayed in this book have a goal in mind, but can have limitless variations, and even entirely new courses can be developed—as long as you have a goal in mind. Use these drills to your advantage and also keep a trained eye out for new drills that may be useful to implement into your own successful agility program.

2

Boxes

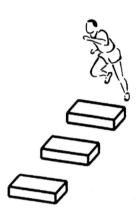

Level I

In/out

Horizontal run around

Run through

Step on/off

Two feet on/over

Forward/backward around

Lateral shuffle around

Offset run around

Stair hop

Level II

Forward/backward

Lateral shuffle

Two-feet jumps over

Jumping jack

Lateral two-feet jump over

Two jumps and shuffle

Star

S forward

S lateral

Star facing in

Star around

Level III

Horizontal boxer

Two-feet lateral jumps over

Horizontal ski jumps

Vertical boxer

Vertical ski jumps

Up and over

Pyramid

Stair hop with turn

Forward jump with a twist

Lateral two-jump run/ backpedal

The boxes used in these drills are standard aerobic boxes. They are 15" x 27" x 6" plastic boxes that can be stacked and still maintain their stability. They are not the aerobic boxes that require risers. These boxes are good because you can jump on, jump over, and run around them. In the diagrams, only five boxes are shown; for the drills, use 10 boxes.

Boxes can be used for both agility and power. For agility, emphasize correct running mechanics, especially the leg drive from the hip flexors. Many young athletes do not have good leg-swing when they run. Boxes emphasize the need to push off, which will help bring the knees up. However, *you must watch their technique*. Some athletes will abduct at the hip, causing their thighs or knees to flair out, instead of using good hip flexors and driving the knee forward. This "puppy on the fire hydrant" stance can cause poor technique.

The second purpose of the box is to develop power. Since power is not the same as true plyometric training, stack the boxes no more than three high. You want the athletes to get the correct technique, so emphasize form, especially the arms. Blocking (the short movement from hips to forehead of both arms simultaneously as you propel yourself up) can increase jumping ability by 10 to 15 percent if done correctly (36). Watch your athletes' technique carefully and see if they are rounding at the back or leaning too far forward at the hips when jumping onto the box. If so, then they are using a box that is too high and are learning poor technique. Research (3, 36) shows that you find the correct box height by having the athlete do a vertical jump. Then, have them step off the box, land, and explode up to their original vertical jump height. Continue to have the athlete move up in boxes until they cannot step off the box, land, and explode to their original vertical jump height. It is better to have them use a slightly smaller box and focus on explosiveness than to use a box that is too high and risk an injury or reinforce poor technique.

Variations

Variations can be made to all the drills to increase the intensity. One variation is using one leg instead of two. You want your athletes to land without wobbling from side to side or having forward lean. These tendencies may mean they do not have the strength or balance to perform the drill correctly and can cause an injury. Going backwards is another variation, but again, the athlete needs good balance and coordination to perform the drill correctly. For progression, have the athletes go through all three levels. Start at level I drills and have them perform them on one leg or backwards. As they become more proficient, then they can move to level II and III with one leg or backwards. Before you try to increase the intensity, make sure they can perform the drill correctly.

Set-up and Format

The purpose of these drills is to teach agility, not conditioning. Make sure you give athletes enough rest after each set so they can fully recover before starting the next set. Use about 10 boxes for agility, with the exception of the star and stair drills, which only use four and five boxes, respectively. The athletes go down one way and stay at that end until it is time to come back. This arrangement ensures that both the right and left legs have a chance to be the lead leg. You may find an athlete can successfully go down the ladder with the right leg leading, and have trouble with the left leg coming back. This problem is not uncommon and is the reason athletes should perform the drills both ways.

Box Placement

The boxes are placed vertically, horizontally, and offset (see Figure 2-1). Each placement has patterns at all three levels, with level I being the easiest, level II moderate, and level III the hardest. When setting up the boxes, you want at least two feet spacing in between each box so that the athlete will have enough room to maneuver around the boxes without hitting them. Set up two rows so that you can accommodate up to 30 athletes per session. For agility, keep it at one box high; for power, never use more than three high.

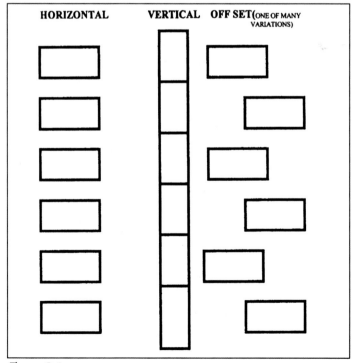

Figure 2-1

Drill #1: In/Out

Objective: To develop feet and quick change of direction.

Description:

- Standing with the first box on his left side, the athlete backpedals down and around the box so he is in between the first and second box.
- The athlete sprints forward so he is at the top of the second box.
- The athlete backpedals down and around the second box so he is in between the second and third box.
- The athlete sprints forward so he is at the top of the third box.
- Repeat.

Coaching Points:

- Make sure the athlete runs all the way to the top of the box.
- Tell the athlete to stay down when transitioning from run to backpedal.
- The athlete should use short, quick steps.

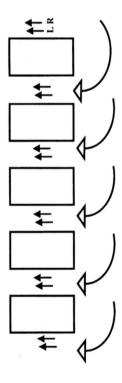

Drill #2: Horizontal Run Around

Objective: To develop balance while running in a turn. The athlete must be able to accelerate and decelerate quickly without losing a step.

Description:

- The athlete is standing on the right side of the box.
- The athlete runs to the top of the box and places his hand on the box as he goes around it.
- He runs to the top of the next box and places his hand on it as he goes around it.
- Repeat.

Coaching Points:

- The athlete must maintain core stability as he goes around the boxes.
- Hips should lower as the athlete decelerates.
- Watch for quality arm action.

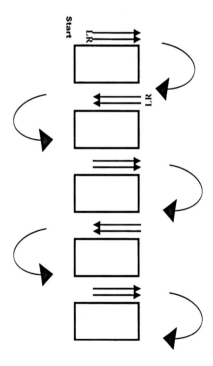

Drill #3: Run Through

Objective: To develop knee lift while running.

Description:

- Standing behind the first box, the athlete runs over the box.
- One foot goes in between each box.

Coaching Points:

- The athlete should lift his knees as he goes over the box.
- Make sure the athlete is using his arms correctly.

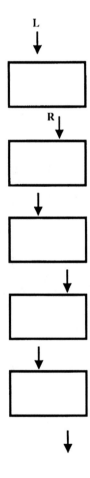

Drill #4: Step On/Off

Objective: To develop fast feet and knee lift.

Description:

- The athlete faces the boxes so his shoulders are parallel to the length of the box.
- The athlete steps on with the left leg, then the right leg.
- The athlete steps backwards and diagonally off the box so he is lined up with the next box.
- The athlete steps up on the second box with the left leg, followed by the right leg.
- If the athlete is moving left, the left leg leads. If the athlete is moving right, then the right leg leads.

Coaching Points:

- The athlete should maintain core stability when moving.
- Make sure he steps on the box with the correct foot (lead leg).
- The athlete should step up on the box so he does not kick it forward.
- Make sure the athlete uses his arms correctly.

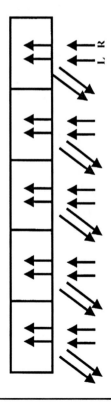

Drill #5: Two Feet On/Over

Objective: To develop triple joint extension and balance.

Description:

- Standing with the boxes on the right side, the athlete jumps onto the first box with both feet.
- Next, he jumps to the right side of the box.
- Then, he jumps left, back onto the second box.
- Repeat.

Coaching Points:

- The athlete should use his arms in an upward motion.
- Make sure he lands without making a thumping sound.
- Remind him to maintain core stability on takeoff and landing.

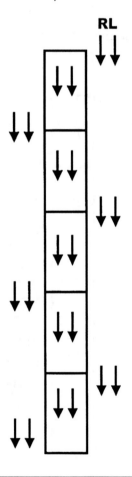

Drill #6: Forward/Backward Around

Objective: To develop forward/backward movement patterns and eliminate false steps during transition.

Description:

- Standing on the right side of the first box, the athlete backpedals past the second box (going around it by about two feet).
- Once he is past the box, he runs forward until he gets around the second box.
- He goes around it and starts to backpedal again.
- Repeat.

Coaching Points:

- Tell the athlete to maintain correct running position when backpedaling.
- Make sure the athlete does not false step as he goes from backpedal to sprint.
- The athlete should lower his center of gravity on transition.

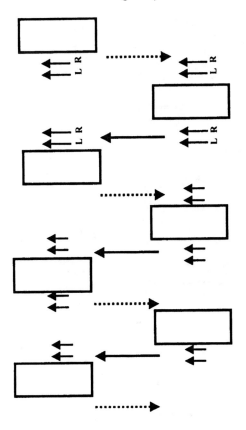

Drill #7: Lateral Shuffle Around

Objective: To develop agility and lateral balance.

Description:

- Facing forward so the box is to the right of him, the athlete shuffles to the left until he gets around it (going around it by about two feet).
- Once he is past the box, he shuffles left until he gets around the second box.
- Repeat.

Coaching Points:

- The athlete should not bend over when transitioning from side to side.
- Remind the athlete to push off with the opposite foot.
- Make sure he does not cross over.
- The athlete should lower the center of gravity when transitioning.

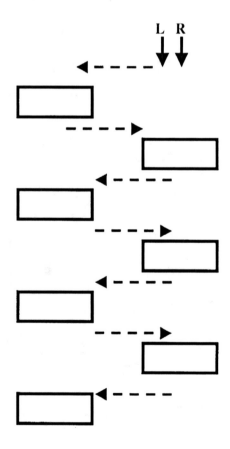

Drill #8: Offset Run Around

Objective: To develop correct body lean when running around a turn and to work on acceleration/deceleration.

Description:

- Facing the coach so the box is to the left of him, the athlete runs forward until he gets around the box.

- The athlete puts his hand on the box, keeping his feet moving, and goes around it so he is facing the second box.

- He runs until he reaches the end of the second box, puts his hand on it, and goes around it.

- Repeat.

Coaching Points:

- The athlete should keep his torso rigid, not bent at the waist, when going around a turn.

- Make sure the athlete uses his arms correctly when running.

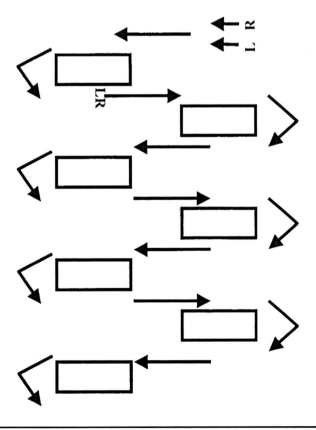

Drill #9: Stair Hop

Objective: To develop short, quick bursts of explosive power.

Description:

- The athlete stands so his shoulders are parallel to the first box, then jumps over it with both feet.
- He lands behind the box, then jumps laterally to his left so he is in the middle of the second box.
- He jumps forward with both feet over the second box, then jumps laterally to his left so he is in the middle of the second box.
- Repeat.

Coaching Points:

- The athlete should not stay on the ground a long time between jumps.
- Watch for correct form on knees and arms.

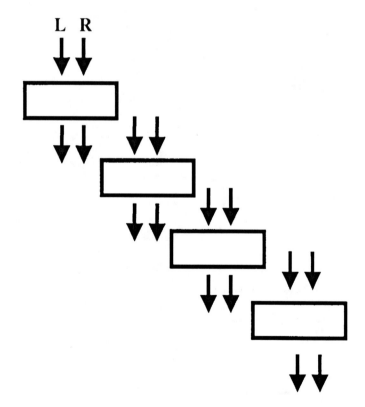

Drill #10: Forward/Backward

Objective: To develop sprinting/backpedaling technique. To teach athletes how to shift their weight while maintaining correct body posture when they change direction and to eliminate false steps.

Description:

- The athlete is standing on the right side of the box.
- He runs past the top of the box (approximately two feet past).
- He backpedals around the box so he is past it.
- Repeat.

Coaching Points:

- The athlete should not stand up when transitioning from forward to backward movement.
- Make sure the athlete does not false step when transitioning.
- Watch for proper arm movement when the athlete is moving.

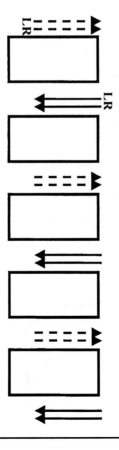

Drill #11: Lateral Shuffle

Objective: To develop lateral movement and the ability to shift weight when moving side to side.

Description:

- The athlete is standing so his shoulders are parallel to the box.
- He shuffles to the left, past the top of the box (approximately two feet past).
- He shuffles around the box to the right so he is past it.
- Repeat.

Coaching Points:

- The athlete should not rise up as he changes direction.
- Make sure the athlete does not cross over his feet.

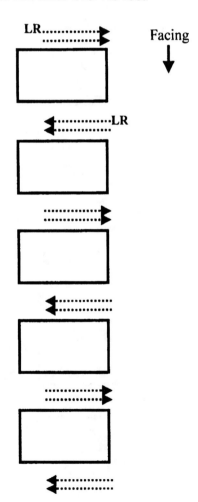

Drill #12: Two-Feet Jumps Over

Objective: To develop balance and explosiveness in the legs.

Description:

- Standing behind the first box, the athlete jumps with both feet over the first box, landing on the ground between boxes.

- Repeat.

Coaching Points:

- The athlete should be under control the whole time.

- Remind the athlete to maintain core stability on takeoff and landing.

- Tell the athlete to use his arms to enhance jumps—not for balance.

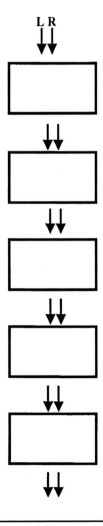

Drill #13: Jumping Jack

Objective: To develop footwork and agility. (This drill is a good warm-up exercise.)

Description:

- The athlete jumps onto the box with both feet.
- He jumps off the box, so the left leg is on the left side and the right leg is on the right side.
- He jumps back onto the box with both legs in the middle of the box.
- He jumps forward and repeats.

Coaching Points:

- Look for good core stability.
- The athlete should use quick feet.
- Remind the athlete to use proper arms action.

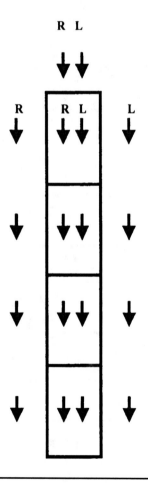

Drill #14: Lateral Two-Feet Jump Over

Objective: To develop forward and backward jumping power and coordination.

Description:

- The athlete faces the boxes so his shoulders are parallel to the boxes.
- He jumps over the boxes with both feet, keeping the shoulders parallel to the boxes.
- He jumps backwards over the boxes, landing so he is lined up with the second box.
- Repeat.

Coaching Points:

- The athlete should stay in proper position when jumping, especially on the backwards jumps.
- Arms are used to enhance jumping—not just for balance.
- Watch for proper knee lift on the jumps.
- The athlete should be facing forward, not diagonal, the entire time.

Variation: If the athlete cannot jump over the box, have them jump on, then over.

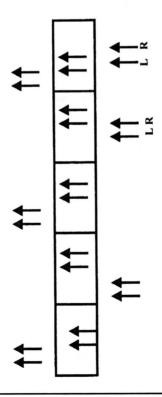

Drill #15: Two Jumps and Shuffle

Objective: To develop vertical power and lateral movement.

Description:

- Facing forward so the box is in front, the athlete hops over the first box, lands on the ground, then quickly hops over the second box.
- He shuffles left until he is lined up with the third box.
- He hops forward over the third and fourth boxes.
- He shuffles to the right so he is lined up with the fifth and sixth boxes.

Coaching Points:

- The athlete should hit the ground and explode quickly to utilize the stretch-shortening cycle.
- The waist should not bend during landing.
- Watch for proper arm movement.
- The athlete should stay low in the lateral shuffle.

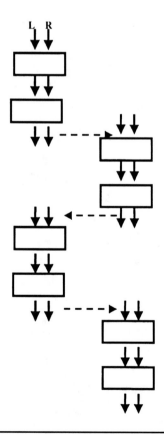

Drill #16: Star

Objective: To develop short, quick jumping skills.

Description:

- Starting on the right side of box 1, the athlete jumps laterally over it.
- He lands with both feet on the left side of box 1, then jumps forward so his shoulders are parallel to box 2.
- He jumps forward over box 2 with both feet, landing in front of it.
- He jumps forward so his shoulders are perpendicular to box 3.
- He jumps laterally over box 3.
- He jumps backward so his shoulders are parallel to box 4.
- He jumps backwards over box 4.

Coaching Points:

- The athlete should not stay on the ground a long time. He should use fast feet.
- Remind the athlete to pick up his knees when jumping.

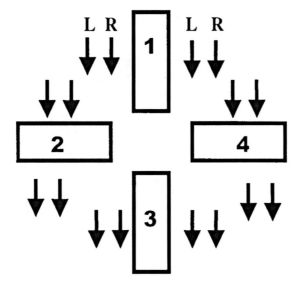

Drill #17: S Forward

Objective: To develop lateral and vertical explosiveness.

Description:

- Standing so his shoulders are parallel to the first box, the athlete jumps with both feet over it.

- He lands behind the box, then jumps laterally to his right so he is in the middle of the second box.

- He jumps forward with both feet over the second box, then jumps laterally so he is lined up with the third box.

- He jumps over the third box, then jumps laterally right so he is lined up with the fourth box.

- Repeat.

Coaching Points:

- The athlete should use short, quick arm movements.

- Make sure the athlete pops off of the ground. He should not stop and reset.

- Knees should be up.

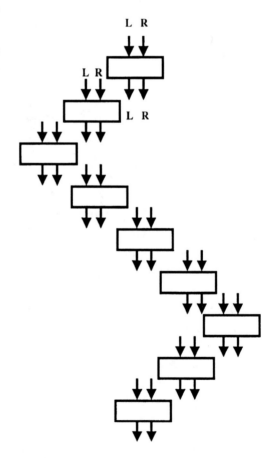

Drill #18: S Lateral

Objective: To develop kinesthetic awareness while in motion. Athletes will move in all directions, focusing on correct movement mechanics, transition, and speed.

Description:

- The athlete stands on the right side so his shoulders are perpendicular to the first box, then jumps laterally with both feet over it.
- He lands on the left side of the box, then jumps forward so he is in the middle of the second box.
- He jumps laterally with both feet over the second box, then jumps forward so he is lined up with the third box.
- He jumps laterally over the third box, then jumps backwards so he is lined up with the fourth box.
- Repeat.

Coaching Points:

- The athlete should be in an athletic position.
- Hips should open when turning.
- The athlete should move slowly with *quality* footwork.
- The athlete should only move as fast as he can correctly.
- The body should stay low while turning.
- Head should move as if on a swivel.

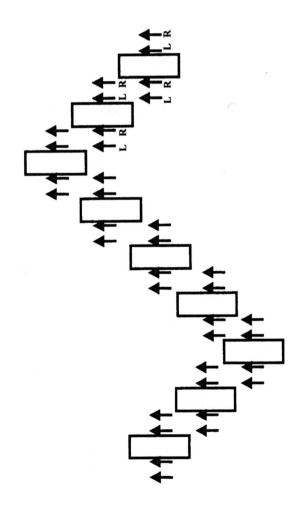

Drill #19: Star Facing In

Objective: To develop balance while moving laterally in a low position. This drill is especially good for wrestlers, football players, or athletes in any combative sport.

Description:

- Starting on the right side of box 1, the athlete jumps laterally over it.
- He lands with both feet on the left side of box 1, then jumps horizontally with a 90-degree turn so his shoulders are perpendicular to box 2.
- He jumps laterally over box 2 with both feet, landing on the left side of it.
- He jumps horizontally with a 90-degree turn so his shoulders are perpendicular to box 3.
- Repeat pattern.

Coaching Points:

- The athlete should stay in the same position as he moves through the entire drill. He should not stand up as he jumps or lands.
- Feet should not cross over.
- Remind the athlete to maintain balance while jumping.
- Make sure the athlete does not lean from side to side.

Modifications:

- Put the boxes closer and have the athletes put their hands on the boxes as they move over the boxes.
- Cue which direction to move.

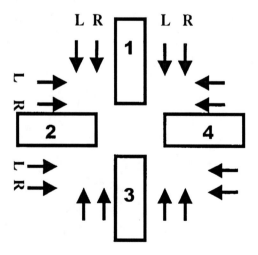

Drill #20: Star Around

Objective: To develop balance while moving laterally in a low position.

Description:

- The athlete starts on the right side of box 1, with hands on the ground in the middle of the boxes.

- He steps off with both feet to the left side of box 1, keeping his hands on the ground.

- He steps off with both feet on the left side of box 2, keeping his hands on the ground.

- Repeat pattern.

Coaching Points:

- The athlete should stay in the same position as he moves through the entire drill. He should not stand up as he jumps or lands.

- Feet should not cross over.

- The athlete should maintain balance while moving.

- Hands do not lift from the ground.

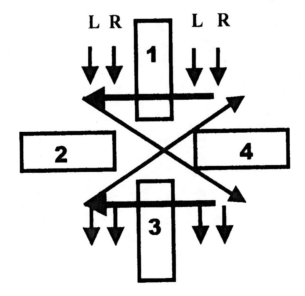

Drill #21: Horizontal Boxer

Objective: To develop one-legged agility, coordination, and balance.

Note: This drill is similar to the jumping jack drill. However, it requires more balance and coordination. The athlete must be able to hop and balance on one leg.

Description:

- The athlete jumps onto the box with both feet.
- He jumps off the right side of the box, landing on the right leg.
- He jumps back onto the box with the right leg, landing on both legs.
- He jumps off the left side of the box, landing on the left leg.
- He jumps back onto the box with the left leg, landing on both legs.
- He jumps forward off the box and repeats the right/left side jumps for each box.
- He jumps onto the next box and repeats the right/left side jumps.

Coaching Points:

- The athlete should maintain proper balance while landing on one foot.
- Arms should be used for upward drive.
- The athlete should jump so he lands on top of the box (if the box moves forward, then his momentum is going horizontal instead of vertical).

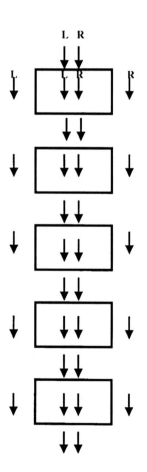

Drill #22: Two-Feet Lateral Jumps Over

Objective: To develop lateral power and balance.

Description:

- Standing with the box on the right side of the athlete, the athlete jumps laterally with both feet over the first box, landing on the ground between boxes.
- Repeat.

Coaching Points:

- Shoulders are perpendicular to the box.
- Arms should assist in upward movement.
- The athlete should land with a stable core.

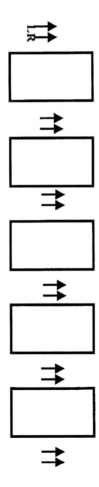

Drill #23: Horizontal Ski Jumps

Objective: To develop two-foot balance and jumping coordination.

Description:

- Standing in front of the box, the athlete jumps with both feet landing on the first box.

- He jumps to the right side of the box with both feet, landing on the ground.

- He jumps back onto the box with both feet.

- He jumps to the left side of the box with both feet, landing on the ground next to the box.

- He jumps back onto the box with both feet.

- He jumps forward off the box onto the ground in front of the box.

- He jumps onto the second box and repeats the sequence.

Coaching Points:

- The athlete should maintain core stability while jumping.

- Watch for proper arm movement.

- Make sure the athlete is balanced when landing.

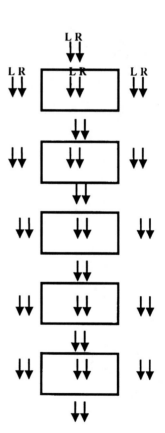

Drill #24: Vertical Boxer

Objective: To develop one-legged agility, coordination, and balance.

Note: This drill is similar to the jumping jack drill. However, it requires more balance and coordination. The athlete must be able to hop and balance on one leg.

Description:

- The athlete jumps onto the box with both feet.
- He jumps off the right side of the box, landing on the right leg.
- He jumps back onto the box with the right leg, landing on both legs.
- He jumps off the left side of the box, landing on the left leg.
- He jumps back onto the box with the left leg, landing on both legs.
- He jumps forward and repeats the right/left side jumps for each box.

Coaching Points:

- The athlete should balance on one leg when he is off the box.
- The athlete should not lean to the side as he jumps.
- Arm action should assist in jumping.
- Make sure the athlete maintains a solid core.

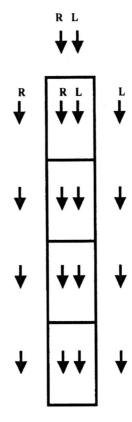

Drill #25: Vertical Ski Jumps

Objective: To develop triple joint extension and balance.

Description:

- Standing with the boxes on the right side, the athlete jumps over the first box with both feet, landing on the left side of the box.
- Next, he jumps with both feet to the right side of the second box.
- Repeat.

Coaching Points:

- Arms should be used in an upward motion.
- Tell the athlete to land without making a thumping sound.
- Make sure the athlete maintains core stability on takeoff and landing.

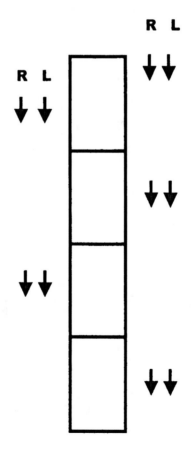

Drill #26: Up and Over

Objective: To develop single-leg explosiveness and balance.

Description:

- Athlete starts with the right foot on the box and the left leg on the ground next to the box.

- He jumps vertically, landing with the right leg on the ground next to the right side of the box and the left leg on top of the second box.

- He jumps vertically, landing with the left leg on the ground next to the left side of the box and the right leg on top of the third box.

Coaching Points:

- The athlete should maintain core stability in the push phase.

- Arms should be used in an upward motion.

- The athlete should push with the foot on the box.

- The waist should not bend during landing.

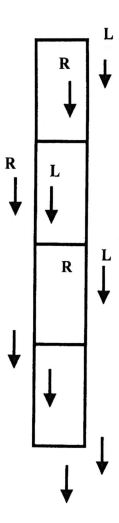

Drill #27: Pyramid

Objective: To develop horizontal and lateral power by using quality triple joint extension.

Description:

- The athlete stands so his shoulders are parallel to the boxes.
- He jumps forward with both feet over the first box.
- He jumps laterally so he is lined up with the second box.
- He jumps forward over the second box, landing on the ground in front of it.
- He jumps laterally so he is lined up with the next box.
- Repeat.

Coaching Points:

- Knees should be up on *all* jumps—not just over the box.
- Look for correct arm action.
- The athlete should not bend at the waist on takeoffs and landing.

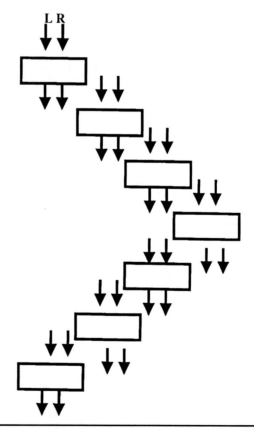

Drill #28: Stair Hop with Turn

Objective: To develop vertical and rotational jumping skills.

Description:

- The athlete stands so his shoulders are parallel to the first box, then jumps with both feet over it.

- He lands behind the box, then jumps horizontally, making a 90-degree turn to his left so he is in the middle of the second box.

- He jumps forward with both feet over the second box, then jumps horizontally, making a 90-degree turn to his left so he is in the middle of the third box.

- Repeat.

Coaching Points:

- The athlete should not overrotate when setting up for the next box.

- Make sure the athlete is set before he trys to jump turn, so he does not twist a knee.

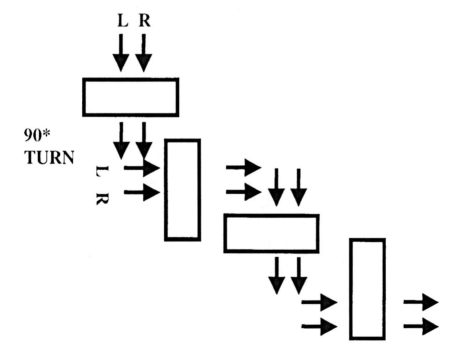

Drill #29: Forward Jump with a Twist

Objective: To develop horizontal and rotational power, balance, and coordination.

Description:

- Facing forward so the box is in front, the athlete jumps over the first box, landing on the ground, then jumps laterally so he is lined up with the second box.
- He jumps forward over the second box.
- As soon as he lands, he jumps vertically and does a 180-degree turn so he is facing the box again.
- He jumps over the second box, then jumps laterally so he is in line with the third box.
- Repeat.

Coaching Points:

- Watch for proper position on landing and taking off.
- Look for quality turns between boxes.
- Emphasize correct arm movement.
- Make sure the athletes use triple joint extension.

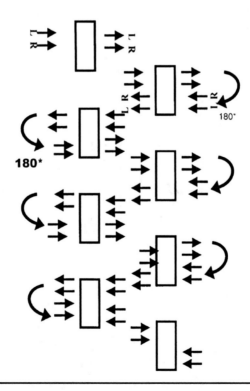

Drill #30: Lateral Two-Jump Run/Backpedal

Objective: To develop power and lateral agility.

Description:

- Standing with the box on his left side, the athlete jumps over the first box, landing on the ground beside it, then jumps over the second box.

- He runs forward until he is next to the third box.

- He jumps with both feet over the next two boxes.

- He backpedals until he is next to the fifth box.

- Repeat.

Coaching Points:

- Hips should not lower excessively on landing.

- The athlete should control the transition from jump to run.

- Make sure the athlete maintains core stability during movement.

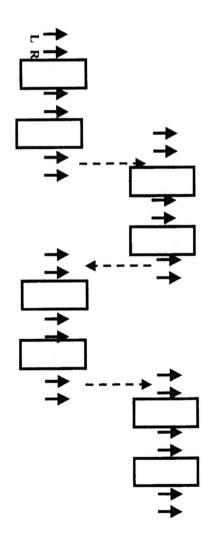

3

Cones

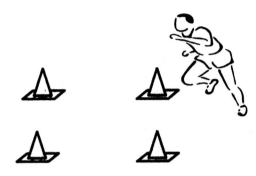

Level I

Forward/backpedal

Forward/backpedal around cones

Lateral shuffle

L course

N drill

Pro agility

Four shuffle sprint

S pattern

Four shuffle ladder

5 – 10 – 5 Race

Level II

Four corner

Four corner around

45 and backpedal

45 and open

Figure 8 with backpedal

Hop with backpedal

Rainbow

T test hop

Triangle reaction cuts

Y react

Level III

Four corner around and back

Around star

Diamond

EKG

Five star

Pyramid

Rainbow react

SPAD

Star multi-direction

Star react

Star react and move

Cone Drill Introduction

Description: The purpose of performing cone drills is to set up courses that mimic specific movements that are performed in sport play. By breaking down movements into single footwork mechanics and performing them repetitiously, motor patterns can be taught and improved performance should be displayed. The coach should make sure that the goal of performing drills is "quality effort"—not quantity. Cone drills should help the athlete learn how to move more quickly and in a more efficient manner, and can also teach body control and decrease injury possibility.

Coaching Points: Make sure that the athlete performs courses at such a rate that mechanics do not break down. Do not progress to higher levels of drills until the athlete shows proficiency with lower level drills. Incorporating lower level drills periodically to maintain basic mechanics can serve as an extension of the warm-up or help as a refresher. Remember that not all athletes will be at the same performance level even though chronological age may be the same. Each athlete will progress at different rates. Make sure to progress athletes according to skill level and not age.

Remember that progression is the key. Make sure that each session has a goal. Try to plan so that one or two aspects of footwork are going to be focused on during each session. For example, on one day of training, focus on drills that require forward movement with stopping and transitioning into a backpedal. Incorporate numerous drills of this nature into one session. Incorporating too many footwork components into one session may lengthen the time it takes for the athlete to master individual skills. When the athletes demonstrate the ability to perform specific movements proficiently, progress into the next level of drills with the same intention as the previous level. Make sure that the duration of each training session allows for proper work-to-rest ratios. If the athletes begin to lose mechanics, they are either getting too short of work-to-rest ratios or they have reached a point of fatigue and conditioning levels have been initiated.

The following drills and levels are designed to help progress athletes through various stages of footwork mechanics. By following the levels and making sure that quality of work is emphasized, your athletes will enhance their ability to move in any and all directions.

Drill #31: Forward/Backpedal

Objective: To develop forward/backward change-of-direction speed.

Description:

- Standing with the cones on the left, the athlete runs to the second cone, breaks down, and backpedals to cone 1.
- He breaks down at cone 1 and runs to cone 3, breaks down, and backpedals to cone 1.
- Repeat.

Coaching Points:

- Is the athlete in correct running position the entire time?
- Does the athlete drop his hips when breaking down?
- Does the athlete stay low in the backpedal?
- Is the athlete using his arms correctly?

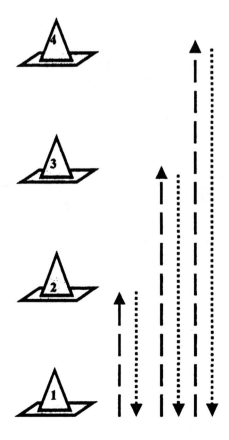

Drill #32: Forward/Backpedal Around Cones

Objective: To develop change of direction while having to avoid obstacles.

Description:

- Standing with the cone on the right side, the athlete backpedals to the second row of cones.
- He goes around the cone and runs forward to the first row of cones.
- Repeat.

Coaching Points:

- The athlete should use peripheral vision to ensure that he does not hit the cones while going around them.
- Watch for correct form when running and backpedaling.
- Make sure the athlete breaks down when changing directions.

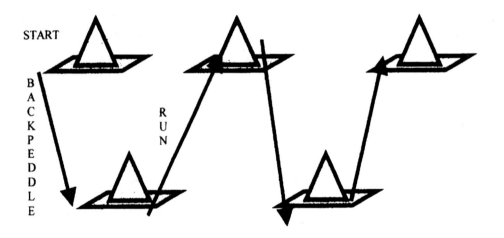

Drill #33: Lateral Shuffle

Objective: To develop lateral movement.

Description:

- Standing so the cone is in front of him, the athlete shuffles laterally to his right around the second cone.

- He goes around the cone and shuffles to the third cone.

- Repeat.

Coaching Points:

- Does the athlete stay in an athletic position while shuffling?

- Is it a shuffle step or a hop?

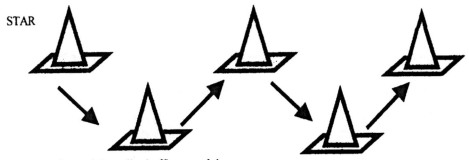

STAR

Facing forward, laterally shuffle around the cones

Drill #34: L Course

Objective: To develop agility.

Description:

- Standing at cone 1, the athlete runs to cone 2.
- He goes around cone 2 to the inside of cone 3.
- He goes around cone 3 and heads back to cone 2.
- He goes to the outside of cone 2 and down to cone 1.
- He runs to the starting line, touches it, and goes back to cone 2.
- He finishes with the last sprint to cone 1.

Coaching Points:

- The athlete should maintain correct technique while going around the cones.
- Make sure the athlete opens up the hips when changing direction.

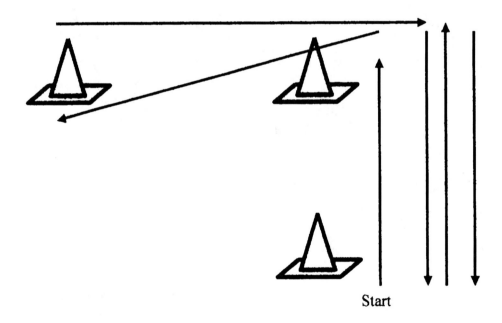

Start

Drill #35: N Drill

Objective: To develop agility and change-of-direction speed.

Description:

- Standing next to cone 1, the athlete runs to cone 2.
- He puts his right hand on the ground and goes around cone 2 to cone 3.
- He puts his left hand on the ground and goes around cone 3 to cone 4.
- He puts his right hand on the ground and goes around cone 4 to cone 5.
- He goes the opposite direction the second time.

Coaching Points:

- Is the athlete keeping good balance as he goes around the cone?
- Did the athlete use correct arm action?

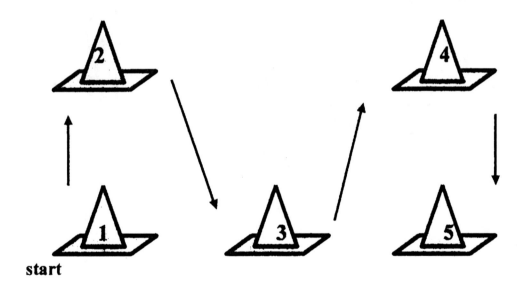

start

Drill #36: Pro Agility

Objective: To develop agility.

Description:

*   Standing with cone 1 in front of him, the athlete opens up and runs to cone 2.
*   He plants with his left leg, opens 180 degrees with his right leg, and runs to cone 3.
*   He plants with his right leg, opens his left leg 180 degrees, and runs back to cone 1.

Coaching Points:

*   The athletes need to turn to the first cone and run, not shuffle.
*   Are the athletes opening up their hips correctly when turning?
*   Make sure the athletes *do not* turn their backs to the cone.

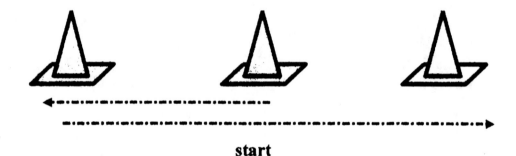

start

Drill #37: Four Shuffle Sprint

Objective: To work on opening up the hips during the transition from a shuffle to a sprint.

Description:

- Standing with cone 1 in front of him, the athlete laterally shuffles to cone 2.
- At cone 2, he opens his left leg 180 degrees, turns, and runs to cone 3.
- Standing with cone 3 in front of him, he laterally shuffles to cone 4.
- At cone 4, he opens his right leg 180 degrees, turns, and runs to cone 1.

Coaching Points:

- Does the athlete raise his hips when moving from a shuffle to a run?
- Does the athlete hop when shuffling?
- Does the athlete open his hips when moving into the run?

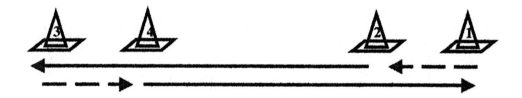

Drill #38: S Pattern

Objective: To develop balance during change of direction.

Description:

- Standing so the cone is on the right side, the athlete runs forward to the next cone.
- He puts his hand on the ground, goes around it, and runs to the next cone.
- Repeat.

Coaching Points:

- The athlete should use correct arm action while running.
- Make sure he breaks down as he gets to each cone.
- Tell him to stay low when transitioning from one cone to the next.
- Have the athletes carry a ball or stick so they have to change arms while going around the cone.

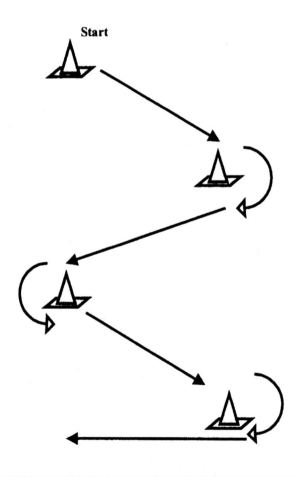

Drill #39: Four Shuffle Ladder

Objective: To develop lateral shuffle.

Description:

- Standing in front of cone 1, the athlete shuffles laterally to cone 2.
- He breaks down, then shuffles back to cone 3.
- Repeat breakdown and shuffle to cones 4 and 5.

Coaching Points:

- The athlete should maintain correct athletic position while moving laterally.
- Make sure he does not bend too far forward at the waist.
- The athlete should maintain balance while breaking down.

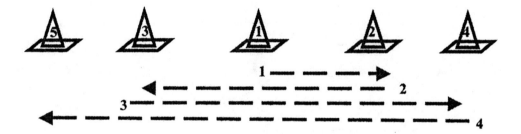

Drill #40: 5 – 10 – 5 Race

Objective: To develop change-of-direction speed while racing another athlete.

Description:

- Both athletes stand facing each other in front of the middle cone.
- Athlete A tells the direction and then says "go."
- Both athletes turn and run to the cone, touch it, then turn and run to the last cone.

Coaching Points:

- The athletes need to turn to the first cone and run, not shuffle.
- Are the athletes opening up their hips correctly when turning?
- Do the athletes go both directions?

A

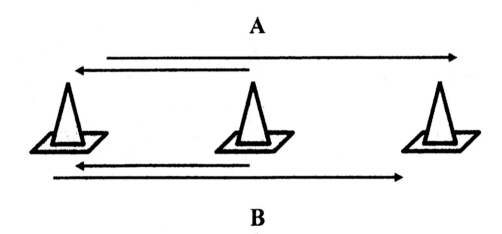

B

Drill #41: Four Corner

Objective: To develop balance during change of direction.

Description:

- Standing so the cone is on the right side, the athlete runs forward to the next cone.
- He cariocas across the top of the cones.
- He backpedals to the next cone.
- He shuffles to the starting cone.

Coaching Points:

- The athlete should maintain stable core while moving.
- He should break down as he gets to each cone.
- He should stay low when transitioning from one cone to the next.
- The coach can use any movement patterns to get around (see variations).

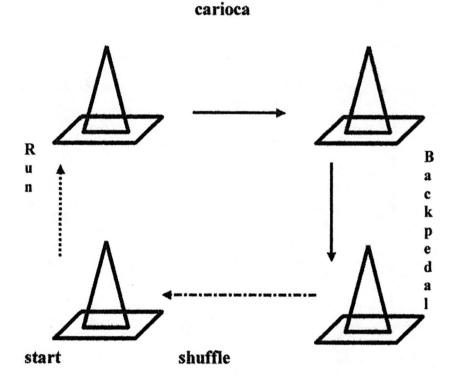

carioca

R u n

B a c k p e d a l

start　　　**shuffle**

Drill #42: Four Corner Around

Objective: To develop balance and coordination while moving around objects.

Description:

- Standing at cone 1, the athlete runs outside and around cone 2.
- He runs back to cone 1 and around it.
- He runs to cone 3, goes around it, and back to cone 1.
- He runs to cone 4, goes around it, and back to cone 1.
- He breaks down at cone 1, opens his hips 180 degrees, and runs through cones 5 and 6.

Coaching Points:

- The athlete should maintain proper body lean while going around the cones.
- Hips should stay low so the feet do not slide out from under the athlete.
- Hips should lower when breaking down.
- Feet should not cross when opening hips at 180 degrees.

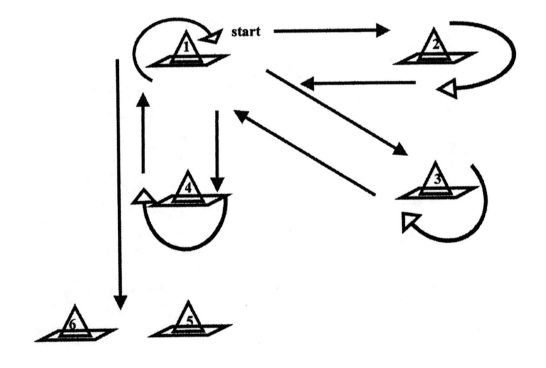

Drill #43: 45 and Backpedal

Objective: To work on opening up the hips when turning.

Description:

- Standing on the starting line cone with cone A in front of him, the athlete runs to cone A, where the coach will indicate a direction to go.

- The athlete opens up his hips and crossover runs to cone B or C (per the coach's instruction).

- At cone B or C, he breaks down and backpedals to the starting line.

Coaching Points:

- Is the athlete in good position as he approaches cone A?

- Is the athlete opening up the hips and using a crossover step when going to cone B or C?

- Does the athlete break down at cone B or C when transitioning into the backpedal?

- Use both verbal and visual cues for the athlete.

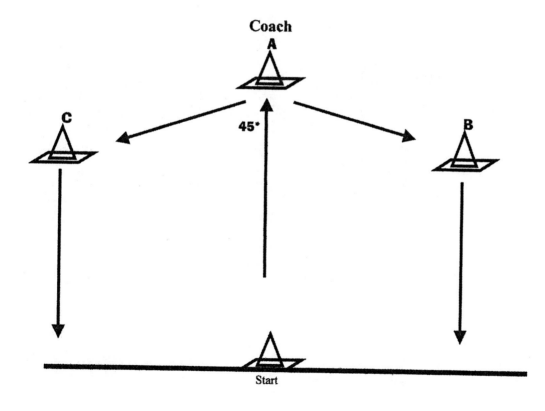

Drill #44: 45 and Open

Objective: To develop correct cutting skills by opening up the hips and breaking down and opening the other way.

Description:

- Standing with the cones behind him, the athlete opens up his left leg to a 45-degree angle and runs to the next cone.

- He breaks down, plants his left leg and opens his right leg 45 degrees, and runs to the next cone.

- Repeat.

Coaching Points:

- Is the athlete opening up with the correct leg?

- Make sure the athlete is not turning his back to you when turning.

- Is the athlete breaking down when he gets to the cone?

- Is the athlete stepping with the correct foot after the breakdown?

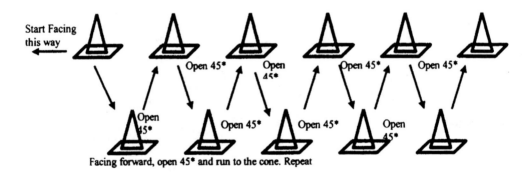

Facing forward, open 45* and run to the cone. Repeat

Drill #45: Figure 8 with Backpedal

Objective: To develop correct running technique as the athlete moves around an object.

Description:

- Standing next to cone 1, the athlete runs to cone 2.
- He goes around cone 2 and runs to the inside of cone 1.
- He goes around cone 1 to cone 3.
- He runs past cone 3, breaks down, and backpedals to the finish line.

Coaching Points:

- The athlete should maintain stable, correct running technique as he goes around the cones.
- Make sure the athlete does not go too wide around the cone.
- Hip level should be kept down in the transition phase.
- The athlete can carry a football or stick while running to simulate game situations.

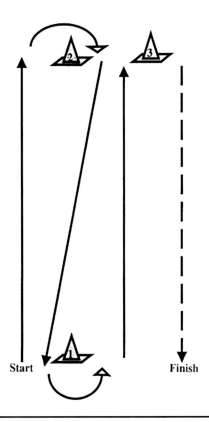

Drill #46: Hop with Backpedal

Objective: To develop power and balance.

Description:

- Standing so the cone is in front of him, the athlete jumps forward with both feet over the first cone.

- He jumps forward with both feet over the next cone.

- He repeats until he gets to the last cone, then shuffles to the right and backpedals to the starting line.

Coaching Points:

- The athlete should maintain his balance while jumping.

- Arms should be used for locomotion, not balance.

- Make sure the athlete breaks down after jumping to get ready for the backpedal.

- Variations can include one-foot hops or lateral hops.

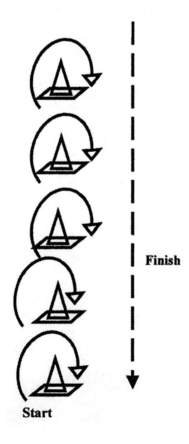

Drill #47: Rainbow

Objective: To develop movement in multiple directions.

Description:

- Standing at cone 1, the athlete laterally shuffles to cone 2, touches it, and shuffles back to cone 1.

- He touches cone 1, then runs diagonally to cone 3. He touches it and backpedals to cone 1.

- He touches cone 1, then runs to cone 4. He touches cone 4, backpedals to cone 1, and touches it.

- Repeat with cones 5 and 6.

Coaching Points:

- Is the athlete in correct position while moving?

- Is the athlete shuffling to cones 2 and 6?

- Is the athlete running to cones 3 and 5?

- Make sure the athlete faces forward the entire time.

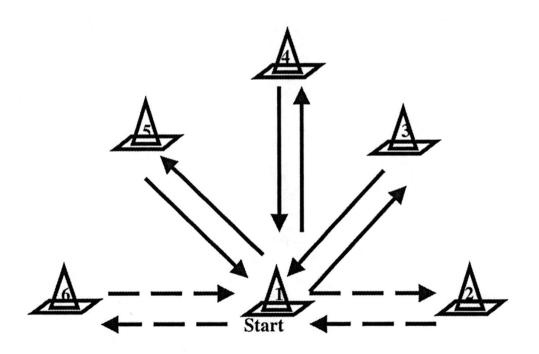

Drill #48: T Test Hop

Objective: To develop balance and power.

Description:

- Standing in front of cone 1, the athlete hops with both feet over cone 1 and cone 2.

- He jumps forward over cone 3, and then laterally jumps between cones 3 and 4.

- He jumps over cone 4, then back between cones 3 and 4.

- He jumps over cone 3, then over cone 5.

Coaching Points:

- Is the athlete using his arms for locomotion and not balance?

- Is body posture correct when jumping and landing?

- Did the athlete maintain stability upon landing?

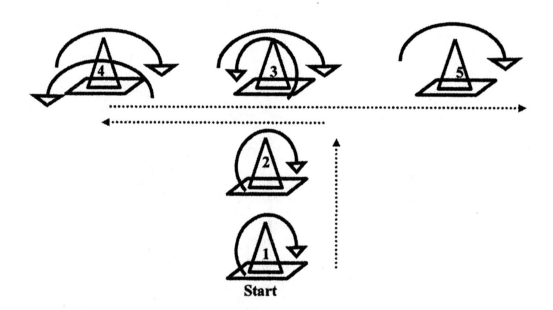

Drill #49: Triangle Reaction Cuts

Objective: To develop cutting and reaction agility.

Description:

- Standing at the starting line, the athlete runs to the first cone, breaks down, and runs to either the right or left cone, depending on the coach's cue.

- He breaks down at the second cone, plants his outside foot, and sprints to the top cone.

Coaching Points:

- Did the athlete break down and use the correct foot to plant and move to the next cone?

- Is the athlete under control as he cuts?

- Use both verbal and visual cues.

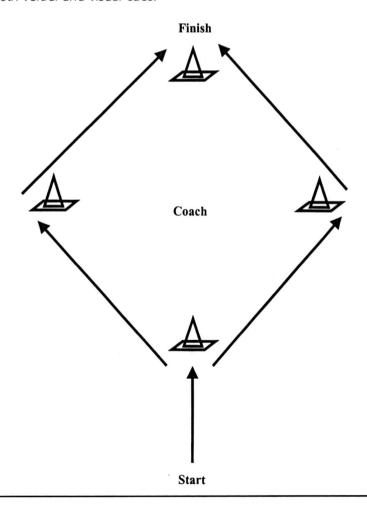

Drill #50: Y React

Objective: To develop correct movement posture after reaction to a cue.

Description:

- Standing next to cone 1, the athlete runs to cone 2.
- He breaks down at cone 2, then moves to cone 3 or 4 after the coach's signal.

Coaching Points:

- Did the athlete break down on cone 2 before reacting?
- Did the athlete take a false step after the signal?
- Use both verbal and visual cues.

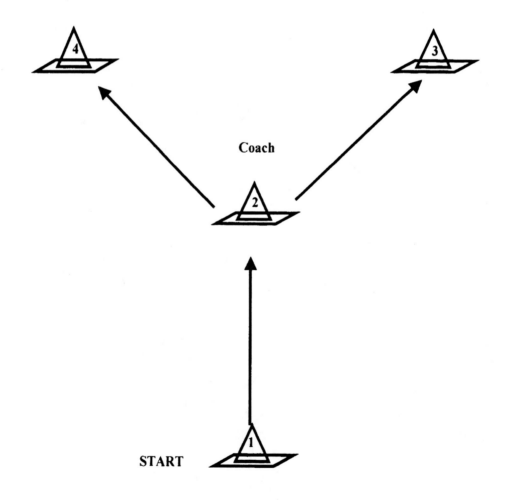

Drill #51: Four Corner Race Around

Objective: To develop balance and coordination while moving around objects.

Description:

- Standing at cone 1, the athlete runs outside and around cone 2.
- He runs back to cone 1 and around it.
- He runs to cone 3, goes around it, and back to cone 1.
- He runs to cone 4, goes around it, and back to cone 1.
- He breaks down at cone 1, opens his hips 180 degrees, and runs through cones 5 and 6.

Coaching Points:

- The athlete should maintain proper body lean while going around the cones.
- Hips should stay low so the feet do not slide out from under the athlete.
- Hips should lower when breaking down.
- Feet should not cross over when opening hips at 180 degrees.

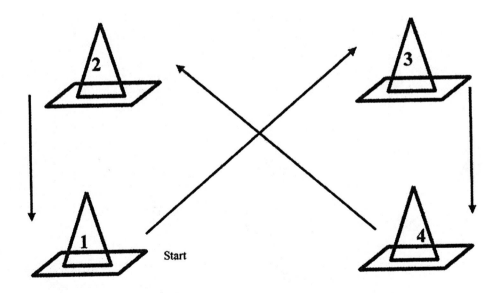

Drill #52: Around Star

Objective: To develop a multitude of movement patterns.

Description:

- Starting at cone 1, the athlete sprints to cone 2.
- He breaks down, and shuffles laterally to cone 3.
- He breaks down, and runs diagonally to cone 4.
- He breaks down, and backpedals to cone 2.
- He breaks down, then cariocas to cone 5.
- He breaks down, opens 45 degrees, and crossover runs to cone 1.

Coaching Points:

- The coach can choose any movement patterns he wants.
- Did the athlete break down at each cone?
- Is there a smooth transition from one movement to another?

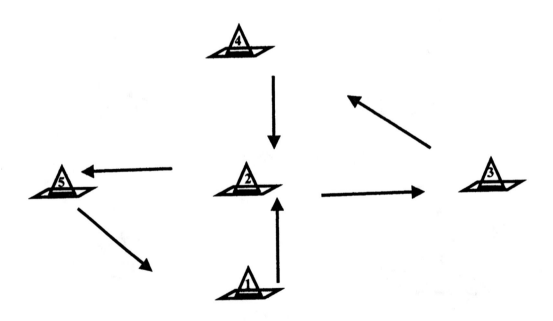

Drill #53: Diamond

Objective: To work on movement patterns in different directions.

Description:

- Standing at cone 5, the athlete runs to cone 1.
- He shuffles to the right and touches cone 2, then shuffles left, back to cone 5.
- He runs forward to cone 3 and touches it, then backpedals to cone 5.
- He cariocas left to cone 4, then cariocas back to cone 5.

Coaching Points:

- The athlete should maintain a stable core while moving.
- Hips and core should me maintained while transitioning from one movement pattern to the next.
- Coach can use any movements the athlete needs to work on.

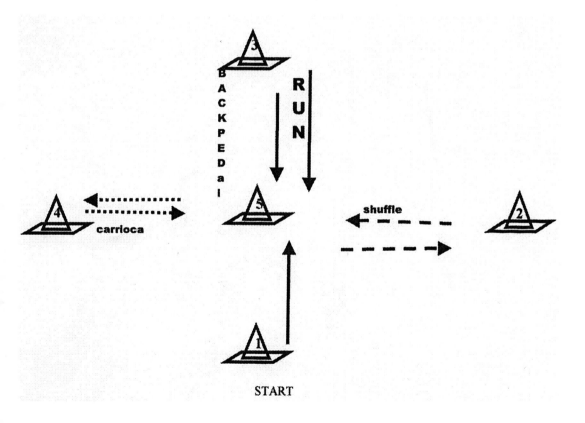

START

Drill #54: EKG

Objective: To teach the athlete how to move laterally, forward, and backward without taking false steps.

Description:

*   Standing so the cones are behind him, the athlete laterally shuffles to the left.
*   After passing the two cones, he backpedals to the next set of cones.
*   He laterally shuffles to the left until he passes the two cones.
*   He sprints past the top cone and then backpedals to the last cone.

Coaching Points:

*   The athlete stays low while transitioning from one movement to the next.
*   Proper running mechanics should be used.
*   The athlete should use peripheral vision.

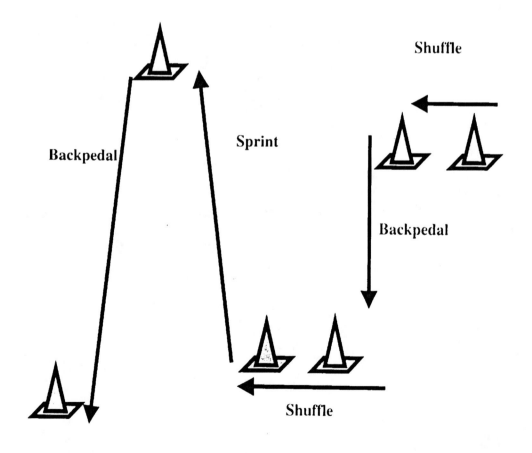

Drill #55: Five Star

Objective: To develop correct technique while running in a diagonal direction.

Description:

- The athlete stands at cone 1, facing cones 2 and 3, then runs to cone 2.
- He backpedals to cone 1, touches it, runs to cone 3, and backpedals to cone 1.
- He opens up his hips 180 degrees so his right foot is pointing at cone 5, performs a crossover step with his left leg, and runs to cone 5. He touches it, opens up 180 degrees so his left foot is pointing at cone 1, performs a crossover step with the right leg, and runs to cone 1.
- Repeat for cone 4.

Coaching Points:

- Is the athlete using correct arm action when running?
- Does the athlete break down when he is at the cone?
- Is the athlete opening up his hips to move in the backward diagonal direction?
- Is the athlete maintaining correct position when transitioning from one direction to another?

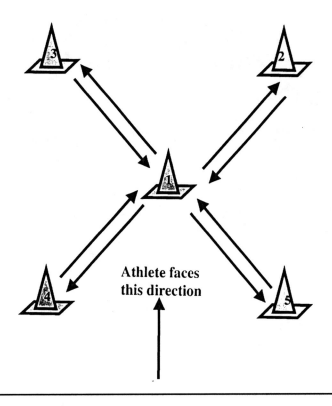

Drill #56: Pyramid

Objective: To develop balance while changing direction.

Description:

- Standing with the cones on the left side, the athlete runs to the top of the first row.
- He goes around the cone and runs back down the second row.
- Repeat.

Coaching Points:

- Is the athlete keeping his feet under him while going around the cone?
- Is the athlete using his arms correctly?
- Is the athlete breaking down as he goes around the cone?

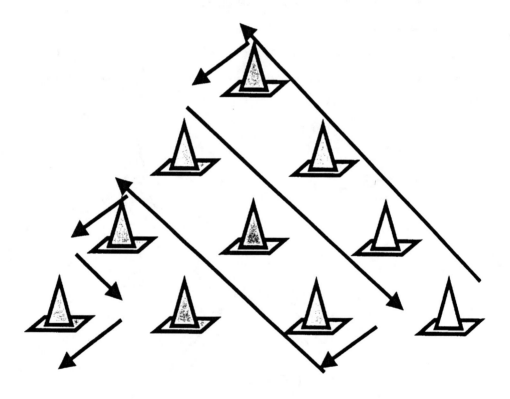

Drill #57: Rainbow React

Objective: To develop movement in multiple directions while reacting to the coach.

Note: This drill is similar to the rainbow drill, except the coach tells the athlete which cone to go to instead of going in a set pattern.

Description:

- Standing at a cone, the athlete laterally shuffles to another cone as indicated by the coach, touches it, and shuffles back to the first cone.

- He touches the first cone, then runs to the next cone as directed by the coach. He touches it and backpedals to the first cone.

- Repeat.

Coaching Points:

- Use verbal or visual (e.g., roll a ball or point) cues to indicate the cone that you want the athlete to go to.

- Do not go in a set pattern. Have the athlete react to your cues.

Coach

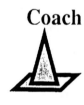

Drill #58: SPAD

Objective: To develop multiple movement patterns with several different pieces of equipment.

Description:

- Standing at cone 1 with the ladder in front of him, the athlete runs through the ladder with one foot in each box.

- He breaks down at cone 2 and shuffles laterally to cone 3, touches it, and shuffles back to cone 2.

- He sprints to cone 4, breaks down, opens his hips 45 degrees, and crossover runs to cone 3.

- He opens up his hips 180 degrees at cone 4 and sprints to cone 1.

Coaching Points:

- Did the athlete use correct form when running?

- Did the athlete break down correctly?

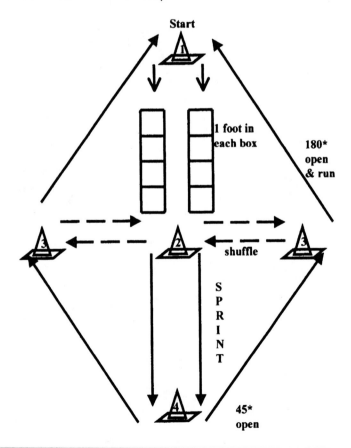

Drill #59: Star Multi-Direction

Objective: To develop balance while moving in several directions.

Description:

- Starting at the first cone, the athlete backpedals to the middle cone.
- He shuffles to the right outside cone, breaks down, opens 45 degrees, and crossover runs to the top cone.
- He breaks down, and sprints to the middle cone.
- He breaks down, and shuffles to the left outside cone.
- He breaks down, and sprints to the starting cone.

Coaching Points:

- Did the athlete keep his eyes on the first cone at all times?
- Was balance maintained when breaking down?
- Did he use correct arm movement?

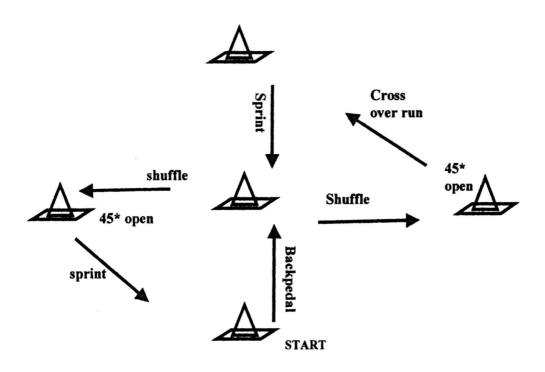

Drill #60: Star React

Objective: To develop balance and strengthen complex leg muscles.

Description:

- Starting at the bottom cone, the athlete runs forward to the middle cone.
- He breaks down, opens 45 degrees with the right leg, and runs to the far right cone.
- He goes back to the start, runs to the middle cone, breaks down, and runs to the top cone.
- From the starting cone, he runs to the middle cone, breaks down, and goes left.
- From the starting cone, he runs to the middle cone, breaks down, opens up 180 degrees, and goes back to the starting cone.

Coaching Points:

- The drill should always start at the bottom cone.
- The athlete should maintain stable core while moving.
- Arms should be used for locomotion, not balance.
- Arms should not swing side to side.
- Tell the athlete to only move as fast as he can correctly.

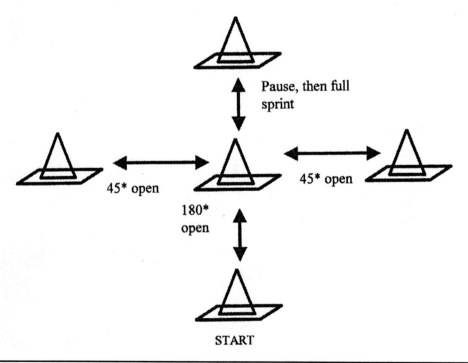

Drill #61: Star React and Move

Objective: To develop proper cutting and running mechanics in an open situation.

Description:

- Standing at cone 1 in an athletic position, the athlete faces the coach and reacts to his command.
- The drill should always start at cone 1.

Coaching Points:

- Start with one cone movement, then progress to two and three movements.
- Check for proper opening of the hips and weight distribution while running.
- Use both visual and verbal cues.
- Remind the athlete to only move as fast as he can correctly.

Coach

Start
Athlete
faces coach

4

Dots

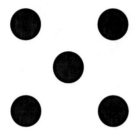

Level I

Alphabet A-Z

Numbers 1-9

The dot drill has been around for a long time and is a favorite of many coaches because it is easy to teach, athletes can grasp the concept quickly, and standardized tests are available so you can compare your athletes to others.

Included in this chapter are some slight modifications to the dot drills and patterns to go with the changes. First, the diagrams include numbers for the dots and between the dots so it is easy for the athlete to understand the pattern. Once the athlete understands the numbering system, you can call out or write down the numbers and the athlete will be able to follow the pattern. The numbering system allows you to make it an open drill and change the patterns so you never have to do the same routine twice in a week. The other modifications that have been made are taking the dot patterns and having the athlete jump rope with them. The traditional dot mat has been expanded to a 5′x5′ (Figure 4-1) area by using agility dots or tape on the ground. Jumping rope is a very good exercise to improve an athlete's agility, balance, and coordination. Using the dot patterns enhances the jump roping exercise by giving athletes a specific purpose. Figure 4-2 shows an example of how the jumps correspond to the numbers.

When maneuvering through the patterns, the athlete should face the same way the whole time to ensure that all the directional movements (i.e., forward, backward, lateral, and diagonal) are covered. If the athlete cannot jump rope and move at the same time, first work on their jump rope skills and then move into the patterns. Always remember: *quality over quantity*.

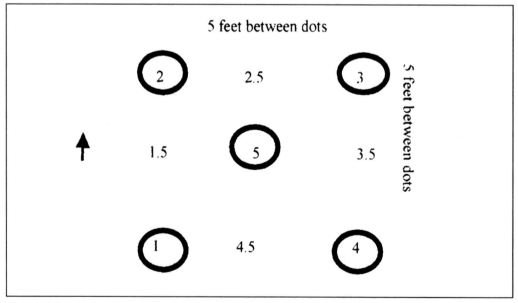

Figure 4-1

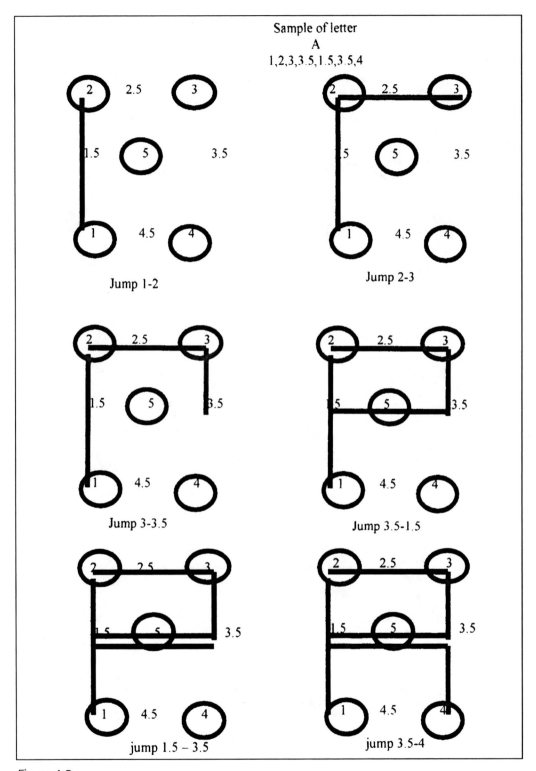

Figure 4-2

Drill #62: Alphabet A-Z

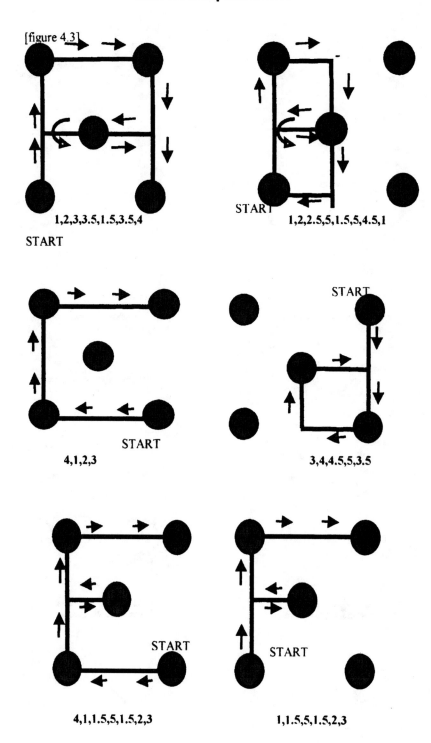

[figure 4.3]

1,2,3,3.5,1.5,3.5,4

START

START

1,2,2.5,5,1.5,5,4.5,1

4,1,2,3

START

START

3,4,4.5,5,3.5

4,1,1.5,5,1.5,2,3

START

START

1,1.5,5,1.5,2,3

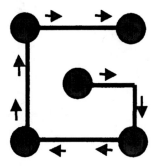

5,3.5,4,1,2,3

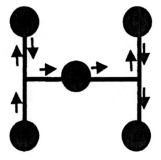

1,2,1.5,3.5,3,4

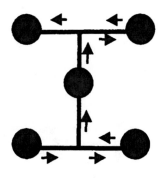

1,4,4.5,2.5,3,2

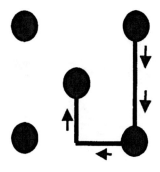

3,4,4.5,5

START

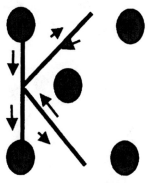

2,1,1.5,2.5,1.5,4.5

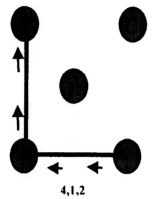

4,1,2

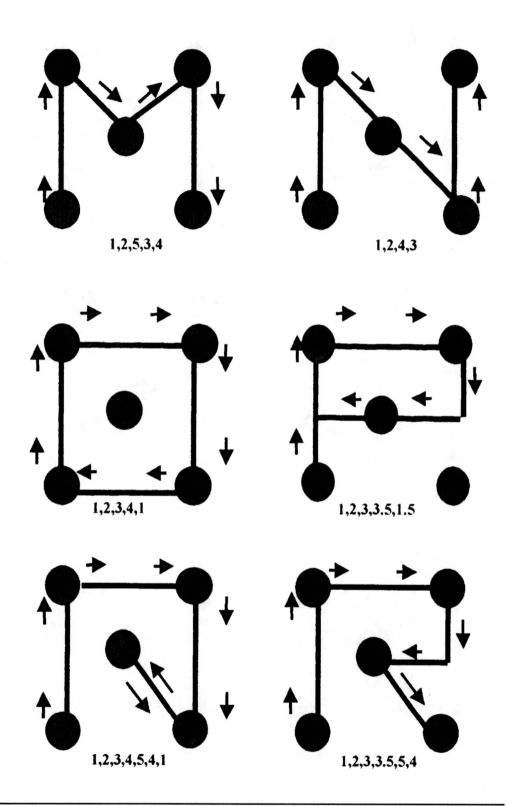

1,2,5,3,4

1,2,4,3

1,2,3,4,1

1,2,3,3.5,1.5

1,2,3,4,5,4,1

1,2,3,3.5,5,4

90

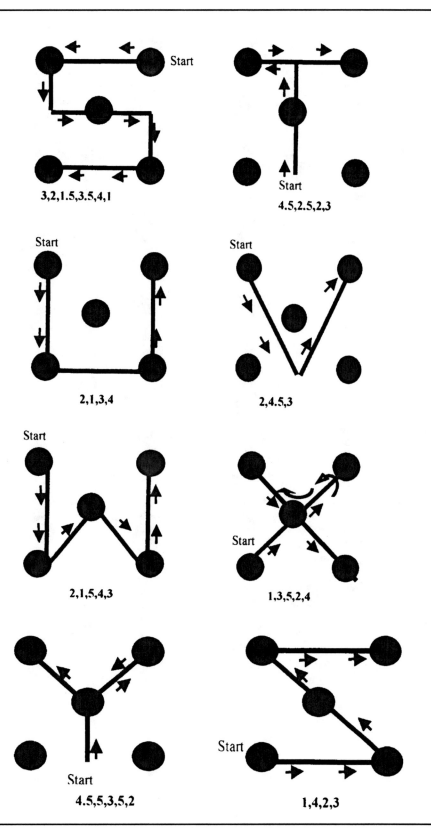

3,2,1.5,3.5,4,1

4.5,2.5,2,3

2,1,3,4

2,4.5,3

2,1,5,4,3

1,3,5,2,4

4.5,5,3,5,2

1,4,2,3

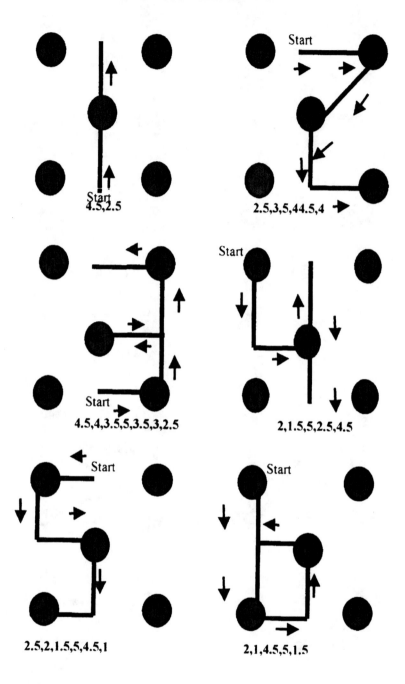

4.5,2.5

2.5,3,5,44.5,4

4.5,4,3.5,5,3.5,3,2.5

2,1.5,5,2.5,4.5

2.5,2,1.5,5,4.5,1

2,1,4.5,5,1.5

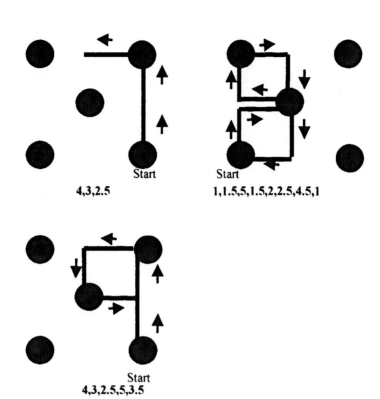

Start
4,3,2.5

Start
1,1.5,5,1.5,2,2.5,4.5,1

Start
4,3,2.5,5,3.5

5

Hurdles

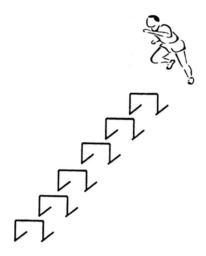

Level I

Double leg hop over

Lateral two-leg hop over

Run through

Level II

Dead leg

Single leg lateral hop over

Scissors

Single leg hop over

Hop shuffle

Supermodel

Level III

Four-corner hurdles

Carioca

Hop/angle run

Hurdles octagon

Hurdle Drill Introduction

Description: The goal of using hurdle courses is to emphasize knee drive while performing movement drills. All of the hurdle drills in this section will include various footwork components that incorporate progressions like all the other drills displayed in the book. As with all drills, you should progress from the lowest level of hurdles until the athlete gains proficiency, then advance to higher levels of footwork components.

Coaching Points: Make sure that knee drive and body control is emphasized during all hurdle drills. This emphasis will force the athletes to pick up their feet and knees. Also, try to have the athlete perform the drills with light and quick feet. All drills should be performed as quickly and smoothly as possible, with technique emphasized. While the athlete is performing each drill, make sure that he maintains good posture and uses proper arm action. Likewise, stress the importance of maintaining a straight upper body when moving forward or laterally. Do not allow the athlete to perform drills while rounding the back.

Drill #64: Double Leg Hop Over

Objective: To develop coordination, power, and balance.

Description:

- Standing in front of the first hurdle, the athlete jumps over it with both feet.
- He jumps forward with both feet over the second hurdle.
- Repeat.

Coaching Points:

- Did the athlete use correct technique when jumping and landing?
- Did the athlete effectively use the hip flexors to get his legs over the hurdles?

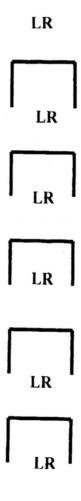

Drill #65: Lateral Two-Leg Hop Over

Objective: To develop lateral coordination, power, and balance.

Description:

- Standing with the first hurdle on his left side, the athlete jumps over it with both feet.

- He jumps laterally with both feet over the second hurdle.

- Repeat.

Coaching Points:

- Did the athlete use correct technique when jumping and landing?

- Did the athlete effectively use the hip flexors to get his legs over the hurdles?

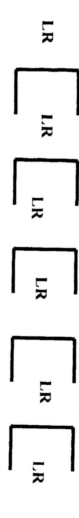

Drill #66: Run Through

Objective: To develop proper leg flexion while running.

Description:

- Standing with the hurdle in front of him, the athlete steps forward with his left foot over the first hurdle.
- He steps forward with his right foot over the second hurdle.
- Repeat.

Coaching Points:

- Did the athlete use correct running form?
- Did the athlete run with good body lean?

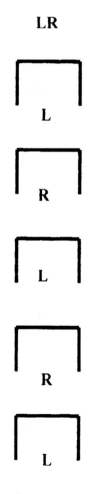

Drill #67: Dead Leg

Objective: To develop proper hip flexion when running.

Description:

- Standing so the hurdle is in front of him, the athlete flexes his left leg at the hip and brings it over the hurdle.
- Keeping his right leg straight, he swings from the hip and moves it so his leg is in between the hurdles.
- Repeat.
- The athlete then performs the drill from the other side—lifting the right leg over the hurdles and swinging the left leg.

Coaching Points:

- Did the athlete use hip flexion and drive the knee up over the hurdle?
- Did the athlete swing the right leg?
- Did the athlete use proper arm action?

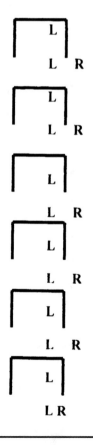

Drill #68: Single Leg Lateral Hop Over

Objective: To develop lateral coordination, power, and balance.

Description:

- Standing with the first hurdle on his left side, the athlete jumps with one foot over it.
- He jumps laterally with one foot over the second hurdle.
- Repeat.

Coaching Points:

- Did the athlete use correct technique when jumping and landing?
- Did the athlete effectively use the hip flexors to get his legs over the hurdles?

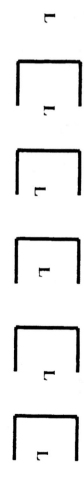

Drill #69: Scissors

Objective: To develop quick feet.

Description:

- Standing so the hurdle is on his right side, the athlete jumps laterally so his left foot is in front of the hurdle and the right leg lands behind it.
- He then jumps laterally so his right foot lands in front of the second hurdle and his left leg lands behind it.
- Repeat.

Coaching Points:

- Did the athlete maintain a straight, upright body position?
- Did the athlete flex at the hips correctly?
- Did the athlete use arms for locomotion, not balance?

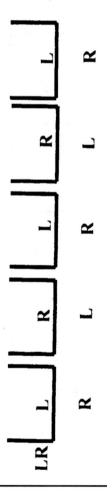

Drill #70: Single Leg Hop Over

Objective: To develop coordination, power, and balance.

Description:

- Standing in front of the first hurdle, the athlete jumps over it with one foot.
- He jumps forward with one foot over the second hurdle.
- Repeat over the remaining hurdles.
- After finishing the course on one leg, the athlete repeats the drill on the other leg.

Coaching Points:

- Did the athlete use correct technique when jumping and landing?
- Did the athlete effectively use the hip flexors to get his legs over the hurdles?

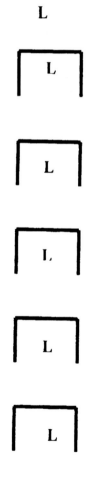

Drill #71: Hop Shuffle

Objective: To develop correct movement patterns after jumping.

Description:

- Standing with the hurdles in front of him, the athlete jumps over the first and second hurdles.
- He shuffles left, then jumps over the next two hurdles.
- He shuffles right, then jumps over the next two hurdles.
- Repeat.

Coaching Points:

- Did the athlete lower the hips on the transition?
- Did the athlete use the arms correctly when jumping?
- Did the athlete shuffle to the next set of hurdles?

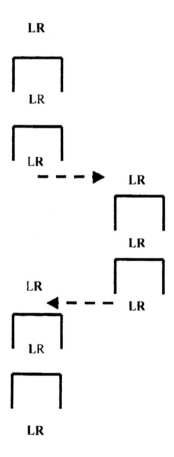

Drill #72: Supermodel

Objective: To develop hip flexibility.

Description:

- Standing with the hurdle in front of him, the athlete steps over the first hurdle with his right leg, placing it on the inside of the hurdle.

- He steps with the left leg on the outside of the second hurdle.

- Repeat.

Coaching Points:

- Make sure the athlete does not use side-to-side movement. The shoulders and hips should stay over the hurdle at all times. Only the feet should be on the side of the hurdle.

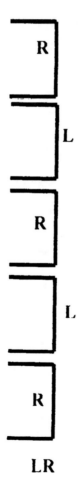

Drill #73: Four-Corner Hurdles

Objective: To develop power, balance, and the ability to jump in any direction.

Description:

- Standing in the middle of the four hurdles, the athlete jumps forward over the hurdle in front of him, then back to the middle.
- He jumps over the left hurdle, then back to the middle.
- He jumps over the right hurdle, then back to the middle.
- He jumps over the hurdle behind him, then back to the middle.

Coaching Points:

- Did the athlete stay facing forward the whole time?
- Did the athlete use his arms for propulsion, not balance?
- Did the athlete maintain correct body position during takeoff and landing?
- Verbally or visually cue the athlete as to which hurdle to jump over.

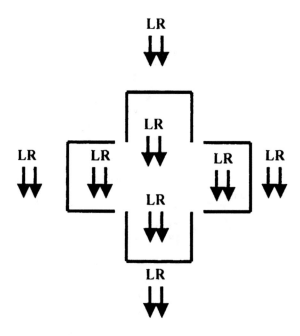

Drill #74: Caricoa

Objective: To develop hip mobility, coordination, and balance.

Description:

- Standing with the hurdles on his left side, the athlete steps over the first hurdle with his left leg.
- He steps with his right leg in front of his left and puts it over the second hurdle.
- He steps with his left leg over the third hurdle.
- He steps with his right leg behind his left and puts it over the fourth hurdle.
- Repeat.

Coaching Points:

- Does the athlete stay facing straight ahead and not turn his body?
- Did the athlete flex at the hip to get the leg over the hurdle?

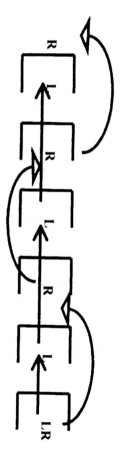

Drill #75: Hop/Angle Run

Objective: To develop a quick transition from running to jumping.

Description:

- Starting in the center of the hurdles, the athlete jumps over the hurdle in front of him, then back to the center.
- He runs in between the front hurdle and the one to his left, then backpedals to the center.
- He jumps over the hurdle to his left and back to the center.
- He runs in between the hurdle to his left and the one behind him, then backpedals to the center.
- Repeat.

Coaching Points:

- Did the athlete take a false step when landing and going into the run?
- Did the athlete use his arms when running and jumping?
- Did the athlete turn to face the correct direction each time?

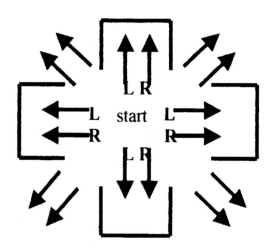

Drill #76: Hurdles Octagon

Objective: To develop power, balance, and the ability to jump in any direction.

Description:

- Standing in the middle of the hurdles, the athlete jumps forward over the hurdle in front of him, then back to the middle.
- He jumps over the second hurdle, then back to the middle.
- He jumps over the third hurdle, then back to the middle.
- Repeat.

Coaching Points:

- Did the athlete stay facing forward the whole time?
- Did the athlete use his arms for propulsion, not balance?
- Did the athlete maintain correct body position during takeoff and landing?
- Verbally or visually cue the athlete as to which hurdle to jump over.

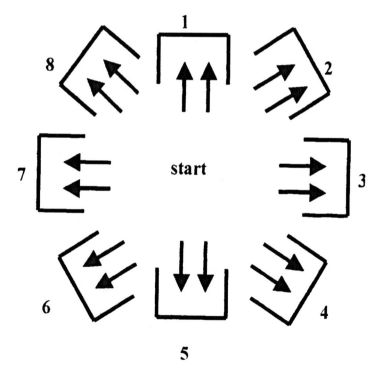

6

Ladders

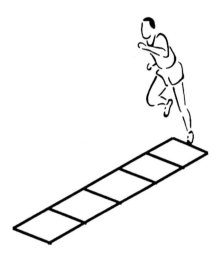

Level I	Level II	Level III
Hopscotch	Carioca	Both in/both out
Jumping jack	Lateral weave with coach	Boxer
Lateral shuffle	Mountain	Icky shuffle
Run through	Step in/step out	In over/down over
Scissors	Supermodel	Lateral single leg hops
	Tree	Right/left leg lead
		Single leg hops
		Snake
		Two-foot split twist
		Weave single leg hops

Ladders

Ladders are a great tool for developing fast feet, coordination, and balance. The ladders that are used in this section are the standard 15′ x 20′ combination plastic and nylon.

To improve running speed, you have to increase frequency (the number of times the feet hit the ground) or stride length (the distance travelled in each step). The ladder enhances frequency by teaching athletes to fire their muscles faster. The drills start out with the basic movement patterns so the athlete is able to focus in on correct running technique, with an emphasis on using the arms properly, flexing at the hips, and not rounding the back. As athletes progress in the patterns, their running movement should be at the unconscious level so they do not have to focus in on their technique and can focus in on the drill and how quickly they can move through it.

With the increase in coordination, the muscles learn how to fire in the most efficient pattern, thus allowing the athlete to become quicker. Coordination also helps an athlete's neuromuscular system adapt to a wide variety of movement situations.

Variations

The nature of the drill is closed (versus open), so to increase the intensity, the athlete must perform the patterns on one leg, backwards, or with limited vision. If you choose to have the athletes do the patterns with one leg, always have them go down with one leg and back with the other to ensure that they are working both legs equally. Before increasing the intensity, make sure the athlete can complete the patterns correctly with good form. Just because he has been doing the same drill for three weeks does not mean the athlete should move on to the next level.

Routine

To increase agility, the athlete must not be too fatigued, so build in rest time between each pattern. Each athletes should go down the ladder and stay at the end until everyone in the group has gone, then come back. This setup allows each leg to be the lead leg, which will develop the athlete's strength on each leg equally. You may find some athletes can go down with the right leg but have a hard time coming back with the left leg leading. This situation is normal and means that the athlete should really focus in on any imbalances he may have.

Teaching New Patterns

When teaching a new pattern, have the athlete walk it and say what each foot should be doing (10). You will be amazed how quickly the athlete will pick up a complex pattern if he says it out loud. You will want to switch up the patterns (using both old and new) so the workouts do not become too repetitive and the athletes do not lose focus on what they are trying to accomplish.

Drill #77: Hopscotch

Objective: To develop quickness and the abductors/adductors of the legs.

Description:

- Standing at the front of the ladder, the athlete hops with both feet so they are next to the first box.

- He then hops into the second box.

- Repeat.

Coaching Points:

- Did the athlete maintain core stability while in motion?

- Make sure the athlete does not go too fast and get out of control or lean his body too far forward.

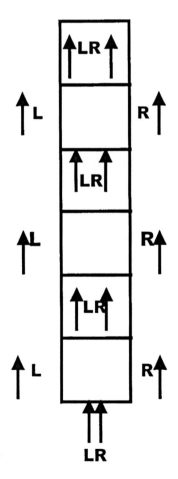

Drill #78: Jumping Jack

Objective: To develop movement in several directions. This drill is a good warm-up because it is easy to learn and gets the athletes moving.

Description:

- Standing at the front of the ladder, the athlete jumps with both feet into the first box.

- He jumps vertically so his right foot and left foot are outside the first box.

- He jumps vertically so his feet end up back in the first box.

- He jumps with both feet to the second box.

- Repeat.

Coaching Points:

- The athlete should maintain upright position.

- The feet should get wider than the boxes.

- Emphasize *quality* footwork.

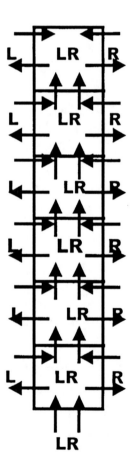

Drill #79: Lateral Shuffle

Objective: To develop lateral movement without crossing the feet, while maintaining athletic position.

Description:

- Standing so the ladder is on his left side, the athlete laterally steps his left foot into the first box.

- Next, he laterally steps his right foot into the first box.

- He laterally steps his left foot into the second box, followed by his right foot into the second box.

- Repeat.

Coaching Points:

- The athlete should not stand up while moving.

- The feet should not cross.

- Make sure the athlete gains ground with his steps.

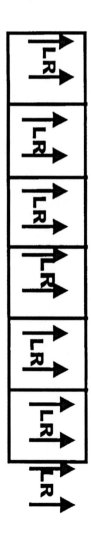

Drill #80: Run Through

Objective: To develop fast feet.

Description:

- Standing at the front of the ladder, the athlete steps into the first box with his left foot.

- He steps into the second box with his right foot, then jumps vertically so his feet are back in the first box.

- Repeat.

Coaching Points:

- Emphasize the importance of using correct running technique?

- Watch the arms for no movement.

- The athlete should pick up the knees and should not drag the feet.

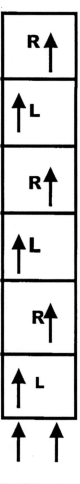

Drill #81: Scissors

Objective: To develop quick feet.

Description:

- Standing so the ladder is on his left side, the athlete jumps so his left foot lands in the first box and his right foot lands behind the first box.

- He jumps vertically and switches his feet so his left foot is on the ground behind the second box and his right foot is in the second box.

- Repeat.

Coaching Point:

- When switching feet in the boxes, the hips should not rotate.

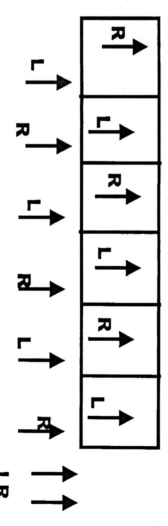

Drill #82: Carioca

Objective: To develop hip flexibility and coordination.

Description:

- Standing with the ladder on his left side, the athlete steps with his right foot in front of his left foot and places it in the first box.

- He steps with his left foot behind his right foot and puts it in the second box.

- He steps with his right foot behind his left foot and places it in the third box.

- He steps with his left foot in front of his right foot and places it in the fourth box.

- Repeat.

Coaching Points:

- Remind the athlete to stay in an athletic position while moving, and not stand straight up.

- Make sure the athlete places the feet in the box.

- The athlete should move slowly with *quality* footwork.

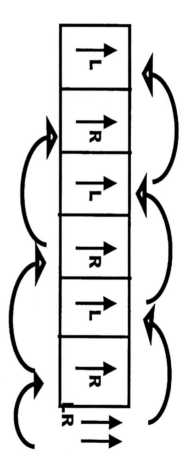

Drill #83: Lateral Weave with Coach

Objective: To develop reaction to an opponent while using correct movement patterns.

Description:

- Standing in the middle box, the athlete moves laterally to the coach's verbal or physical cue.

Coaching Points:

- Emphasize the importance of maintaining athletic position while moving laterally.
- The feet should not cross.
- Make sure the athlete does not stand up when transitioning from forward to backward movement.
- Watch for false steps.

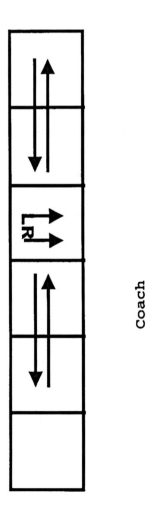

Drill #84: Mountain

Objective: To work on fast feet and lateral movement. The athlete will be able to eliminate false steps when moving forward, backward, and laterally.

Description:

- Standing so the ladder is in front of him, the athlete steps with his left foot, then his right foot, into the first box.

- He steps with the left foot, then the right foot, in front of the first box.

- He steps diagonally backwards with the left foot, then the right foot, into the second box.

- He steps diagonally backwards with the left foot, then the right foot, behind the third box.

- He steps diagonally forward with both feet into the fourth box.

- Repeat.

Coaching Points:

- Make sure the athlete does not false step (i.e., when moving forward, he should not step back, then forward).

- Hips should stay low the entire time.

- The athlete should move slowly with quality footwork.

- Remind the athlete to only move as fast as he can correctly.

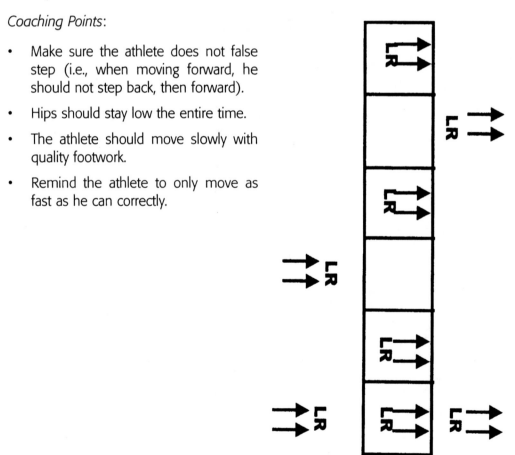

Drill #85: Step In/Step Out

Objective: To develop lateral, backward, and forward movement patterns.

Description:

- Standing so the ladder is on his left side, the athlete laterally steps his left foot in front of the first box.

- He then laterally steps the right foot into the first box.

- He steps the left foot behind the second box, followed by the right foot into the second box.

- He steps the left foot in front of the third box.

- He steps the right foot laterally into the third box.

- Repeat.

Coaching Points:

- The athlete should move backwards without turning the head back to see the feet.

- Does the athlete step with the correct foot in the correct direction?

- Weight should shift weight when changing directions.

- Make sure the athlete pushes off with the correct foot.

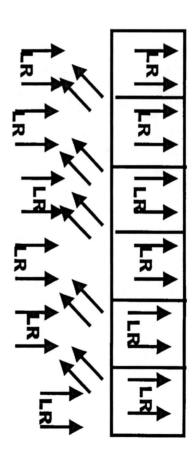

Drill #86: Supermodel

Objective: To improve hip flexibility and hip flexors and to teach leg drive.

Description:

- Standing so the ladder is in front of him, the athlete steps with his right foot and places it on the outside of the first box.
- He steps with his left foot and puts it in the second box.
- He steps with his right foot and places it on the outside of the third box.
- He steps with his right foot and places it in the fourth box.
- Repeat.

Coaching Points:

- The athlete should stand tall when moving (strong core).
- Feet should be in or next to the boxes so hip flexibility is being stressed.
- Make sure the athlete does not move side to side.
- The shoulders and hips should stay forward with lateral movement.

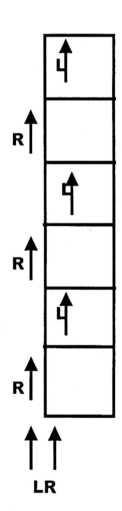

Drill #87: Tree

Objective: To develop kinetic awareness of the feet while moving in a variety of directions.

Description:

- Standing at the front of the ladder with the feet at least shoulder-width apart, the athlete jumps with both feet into the first box.

- He jumps his left foot to the left side of the box and his right foot to the right side of the first box.

- He jumps with both feet into the second box.

- He jumps with the left foot to the left side of the second box and the right foot to the right side of the second box.

- Repeat.

Coaching Points:

- The athlete should maintain correct body position while jumping.

- Feet should move in the correct direction.

- The athlete should move slowly with *quality* footwork.

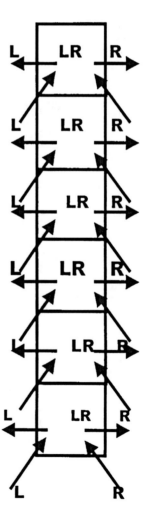

Drill #88: Both In/Both Out

Objective: To develop quick feet. The athlete will learn how to move with the correct foot in the correct direction.

Description:

- Standing at the front of the ladder, the athlete steps the left foot to the left side of the first box and the right foot to the right side of the first box.

- He steps the left foot into the first box and the right foot into the first box.

- He steps the left foot to the left of the second box and the right foot to the right side of the second box.

- Repeat.

Coaching Points:

- The athlete should maintain a stable core.

- Are the feet in correct position?

- Make sure the athlete does not hop.

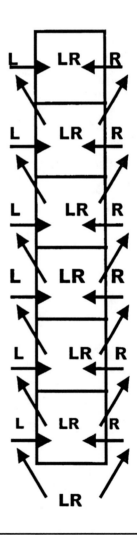

Drill #89: Boxer

Objective: To develop balance and the ability to shift weight while in motion without excessive leaning of the body.

Description:

- Standing at the front of the ladder, the athlete jumps with both feet into the first box.
- He jumps vertically so the right foot is on the outside of the first box and the left foot is in the air.
- He jumps back to the first box with both feet on the ground.
- He jumps vertically so the left foot is on the outside of the first box and the right foot is in the air.
- He jumps vertically so both feet are back in the first box.
- He jumps forward with both feet into the second box.
- Repeat.

Coaching Points:

- The athlete should be able to balance on one leg when landing.
- Can the athlete correctly follow the pattern?
- Does the athlete jump and land on one leg while maintaining stability?
- The foot that is over the box should be lifted, while the other foot is on the ground.

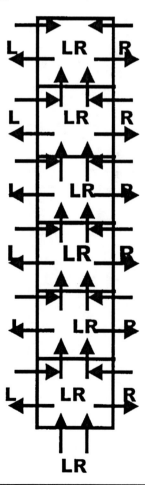

Drill #90: Icky Shuffle

Objective: To develop single leg balance and quick feet.

Description:

- Standing at the front of the ladder, the athlete hops with both feet so they are next to the first box.
- He hops into the second box.
- Repeat.

Coaching Points:

- The athlete should not lean or bend while moving laterally.
- Emphasize the importance of *quality* footwork.
- Make sure the athlete balances on the outside foot.

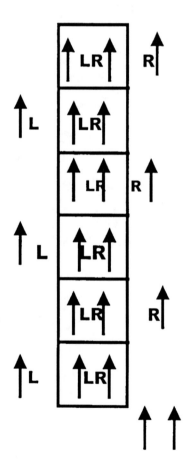

Drill #91: In Over/Down Over

Objective: To develop quick feet and to move in specific patterns so the athlete will eliminate false steps.

Description:

- Standing with the ladder on the left side, the athlete laterally steps with his left foot in the first box, then his right foot in the first box.
- He steps backwards with the left foot so it is behind the first box.
- He steps backwards with the right foot so it is behind the first box.
- He steps laterally so the left foot is behind the second box, followed by the right foot.
- He steps forwards with the left foot so it is in the second box, followed by the right foot.
- He steps laterally so the left foot is in the third box, followed by the right foot.
- Repeat.

Coaching Points:

- The athlete should move in the correct pattern to develop footwork.
- Make sure the athlete does not use any false steps.
- The athlete should move slowly with *quality* footwork.

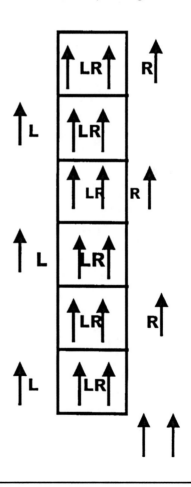

Drill #92: Lateral Single Leg Hops

Objective: To develop balance and strengthen complex leg muscles.

Description:

- Standing so the ladder is on the left side, the athlete laterally jumps with the left foot into the first box.
- He laterally jumps with the left foot into the second box.
- Repeat.

Coaching Points:

- The athlete should maintain a stable core while moving.
- The arms should be used for locomotion, not balance.
- The arms should not swing side to side.
- The athlete should only move as fast as he can correctly.

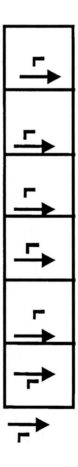

Drill #93: Right/Left Leg Lead

Objective: To develop lower body coordination by having the legs going in different directions simultaneously.

Description:

- Standing so the ladder is on the left side, the athlete laterally steps the left foot in front of the first box.

- He then laterally steps the right foot into the first box.

- He steps the left foot behind the second box, followed by the right foot into the second box.

- He steps the left foot in front of the third box.

- He steps the right foot laterally into the third box.

- Repeat.

- Coming back, the right foot is out of the box and the left leg is in the box.

Coaching Points:

- The lead leg is always out of the box (in front or behind).

- The trail leg is always in the box.

- The athlete should not turn the hips as he switches legs.

- The athlete should balance on one foot while moving.

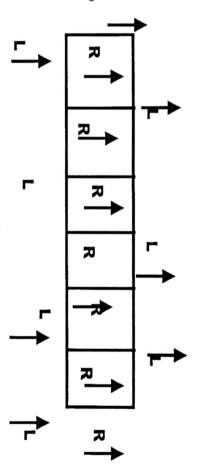

Drill #94: Single Leg Hops

Objective: To develop balance and strengthen complex leg muscles.

Description:

- Standing so the ladder is in front of him, the athlete jumps with the left foot into the first box.
- He jumps with the left foot into the second box.
- Repeat.

Coaching Points:

- The athlete should maintain a stable core while moving.
- The arms should be used for locomotion, not balance.
- The arms should not swing side to side.
- The athlete should only move as fast as he can correctly.

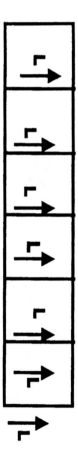

Drill #95: Snake

Objective: To develop hip mobility and quick feet and to work on rotation of the whole body.

Description:

- Standing at the front of the ladder, the athlete jumps with both feet so the left foot lands in the first box and the right foot lands next to the first box.

- He jumps vertically and twists 90 degrees so the right foot is in the second box and the left foot is in the first box.

- He jumps vertically and twists 90 degrees so the left foot is next to the second box and the right foot is in the second box.

- He jumps vertically and twists 90 degrees so the left foot is in the third box and the right foot is in the second box.

- He jumps vertically and twists 90 degrees so the left foot is in the third box and the right foot is on the outside of the third box.

- Repeat.

Coaching Points:

- The athlete should maintain balance while turning.

- Make sure the athlete stays focused so he is not just jumping around.

- Remind the athlete to stay in an athletic position the whole time.

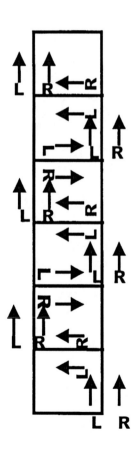

Drill #96: Two-Foot Split Twist

Objective: To develop rotational movement and lower body coordination.

Description:

- Standing so the ladder is in front of him, the athlete jumps with both feet into the second box.

- He jumps vertically and rotates to the right so the right foot lands in box 1 and the left foot lands in box 3.

- He jumps and rotates to the left so both feet land in box 4.

- He jumps and rotates right so the right foot lands in box 3 and the left foot lands in box 5.

- Repeat.

Coaching Points:

- The athlete should be in an athletic position while jumping.

- The athlete should use a short, quick rotational jump.

- The arms should be used for propulsion, not for balance.

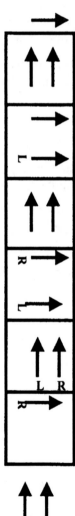

Drill #97: Weave Single Leg Hops

Objective: To develop balance and kinetic awareness while in motion. The athletes will develop single leg strength.

Description:

*   Standing so the ladder is on the right side, the athlete laterally jumps with the left foot into the first box.
*   He laterally jumps with the left foot so it lands to the right of the second box.
*   He laterally jumps with the left foot so it lands in the third box.
*   He laterally jumps with the left foot so it lands to the left of the fourth box.

Coaching Points:

*   The athlete should be in an athletic position.
*   The athlete should keep the hips low by bending at the knees.
*   The arms should be used for propulsion, not as a balancing tool.

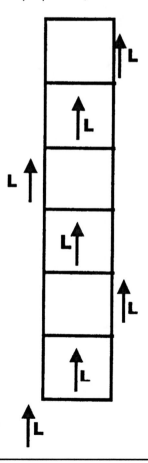

7

Open Drills

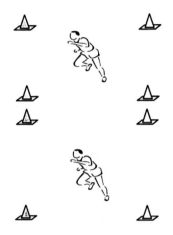

Level III

Box react

Diamond reaction

Octagon

Triangle reaction

Open courses are characterized by not having a definite ending or predictable pattern. Unlike a closed course (such as cone drills), where a specific pattern is followed, open courses are the most specific and also the most demanding of agility drills. The goal of performing open course drills is to create an atmosphere where the athlete must make decisions while in motion. In this atmosphere, the athlete must be able to display superior body control and reactive skills. Thus, all open course drills are characterized as level III drills.

Open course drills use visual or audio cues to indicate changes in direction or footwork components. An example of a visual cue might be a coach simply using hand signals to tell the athlete to change directions. Likewise, an audio cue may be something as simple as the use of a whistle or as complex as giving verbal direction changes. Either way, the athlete must learn to process information while in motion and make fluent changes in direction or footwork.

Closed courses can be converted to open courses by adding open course properties. An example would be to perform a T-drill and have a coach stand at the middle cone of the "T" and give directional or verbal cues when the athlete reaches the middle cone. This simple addition is a good method of introducing the open course method to your athletes.

Coaching Points: Make sure that your athletes can perform nearly all footwork components proficiently before introducing open courses. The addition of information processing while in motion requires the athlete to have quality footwork and also a high amount of body control with regards to upper and lower body mechanics to be able to perform open courses. As stated previously, begin introducing open courses by modifying closed courses with both visual and audio cues before performing any open course drills.

If the athlete has shown quality footwork and demonstrates superior body control but cannot maintain these qualities in open courses, continue to perform high level closed course drills until the athlete can learn to process information and react to cues more effectively. Make sure when open courses are introduced that progression is still the key. Begin with performing the drills that require the least amount of directional changes and also the least amount of footwork components before advancing to the most complex drills.

Conclusion

The following open drills are examples of drills that the authors have found to be effective for enhancing an athlete's performance. Although these drills require a high amount of skill, proper footwork and body positioning must always be emphasized. Studying movements in respective sports can help you develop limitless numbers of open course drills. Make sure that, as a coach, you follow simple guidelines and are creative with drills that may benefit your athletes in the use of open courses. Open course drills can add a fun and competitive atmosphere to your daily training sessions that traditional closed courses do not offer.

Drill #98: Box React

Objective: To develop reaction to another player.

Description:

- Standing on the starting spot, athlete A moves to one of the four cones in his box and then back to the center spot.

- Athlete B must follow athlete A to whichever cone he goes to, then try to beat him back to the center spot.

- Athlete A goes first four times, then switches with athlete B.

Coaching Points:

- Was athlete B able to react to athlete A?

- Did athlete B turn his back on athlete A?

- Was good movement technique used?

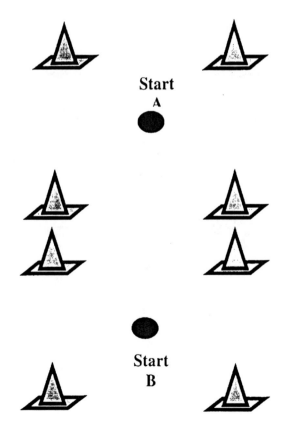

Drill #99: Diamond Reaction

Objective: To develop reaction speed and movement in multiple planes.

Description:

- Standing in the center of the diamond, the coach will call a number and the athlete must move to the cone, touch it, and move back to the starting position.

Coaching Points:

- Can the athlete take a first step without false stepping?
- Did the athlete face the coach the entire time without turning his back to the coach?

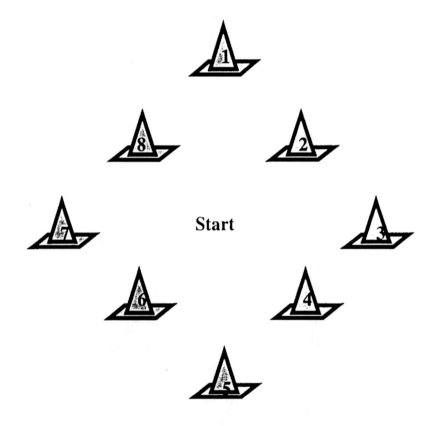

Drill #100: Octagon

Objective: To develop reactive speed in movement.

Description:

- Lay eight pieces of PVC pipe on the ground in the shape of an octagon. Write the numbers 1 through 8 on the pieces of pipe.

- Standing in the center of the octagon, the athlete jumps over the pipe of the number the coach commands.

Coaching Points:

- Can the athlete react to your command or does he have to look at the number, then move?

- Did the athlete jump to the correct number?

- Have the athlete use one leg as a variation.

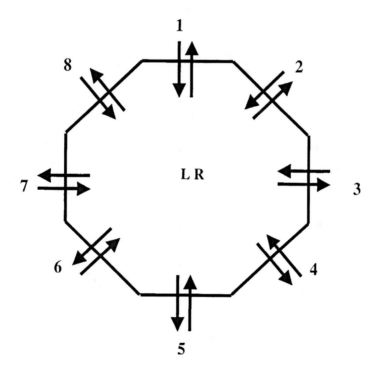

Drill #101: Triangle Reaction

Objective: To develop balance and reaction when jumping in multiple directions.

Description:

- The athlete begins by standing in the middle of the triangle. After the coach's command, the athlete jumps into the numbered triangle, then over the line and back into the numbered triangle.

Coaching Points:

- Did the athlete have to look before jumping, or can he react to your command immediately?
- Did the athlete use correct form when jumping?
- Can the athlete keep up with your cadence?

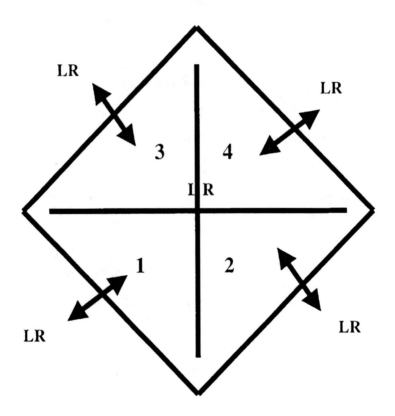

More Open Course Drills

Forward-to-backpedal

Straight stops

Open and closed stops

Mirroring drills

Forward-to-backpedal

Mirroring boxes

- Running

- Forward-to-backpedal

- Run, shuffle, and backpedal

Shuffling

Chase drills

Five points

Ball drops

Standing

Kneeling

Lying

Crazy ball drops

Visual cueing

T-test

Shuffle ladder

Rainbow

Diamond drill

Reaction drill

Audio cueing

T-test

Rainbow

Diamond

Mirroring Drills

Forward-to-Backpedal

The first step in teaching open course forward-to-backpedal is to teach straightforward, open, and closed starts and stops. These terms refer to the body positioning during the transition phase of moving from forward movement to backward movement and vice versa. All stops should be taught with both left and right feet. Straightforward stops are stops in which the athlete will stop with the body remaining square or straightforward. Open and closed stops are both performed by the athlete rotating at the hips and stopping with the body turned laterally. From this position, the athlete drives off laterally and rotates the body back to the squared-up position. For example, when the athlete runs forward and stops on the right foot by turning laterally, the hips are in a closed position. When the athlete transitions from this position by squaring up the hips and upper body, the next stop on the right foot will be an open stop because the hips will rotate in the opposite direction. These types of stops are the most basic forms that are seen in sport.

Have the athlete begin by combining three to five forward-to-backpedaling sequences using all variations of stops and also with both left- and right-footed stops. When the athlete can perform all variations on both feet with good technique and body positioning, begin to add verbal or visual cueing. Verbal cues are recommended to indicate the use of the right or left foot and to specify the type of stopping mechanics that will be used. Using these verbal cues will ensure that the athlete becomes comfortable with starting and stopping on both feet and will enhance acceleration and deceleration capabilities.

When the athlete shows quality footwork and can react effectively to both verbal and visual cues, move on to the final progression of the forward-to-backpedal open course—the mirror drill. In this drill, two athletes will line up 5 to 10 yards apart while facing each other. One of the athletes will be in control, sometimes called the "rabbit." The rabbit will determine all transitions from forward-to-backpedal and the other athlete must attempt to make transitions as quickly as possible following every transition of the rabbit. Have the athletes perform 5 to 10 direction changes and then switch roles.

Coaching Points:

- Make sure that the athlete can perform sound mechanics using both feet before attempting the mirroring drill.

- Enforce quality mechanics before quantity of movements.

- If the athletes cannot demonstrate left- and right-foot starts and stops, then improving those skills should be the first priority.

- All open drills can be the truest form of agility. The athletes can create a competitive atmosphere with the mirror drills. This competitiveness can be added to the drills and serve as a great training atmosphere. Use these drills to enhance your athletes' focus as well as their footwork.

Boxes

The object of the box drills is to have the athlete react much like the mirroring drill for the forward-to-backpedal, except the athletes will attempt to mirror each other in a box-style format. The athletes will face each other in each of their boxes and one athlete will have control or be the "rabbit" again. The athlete with control will run from the center of the box to any of the perimeter cones and return to the center. The athlete that is mirroring runs to the corresponding cone in his own box. As soon as the rabbit reaches the center, he can run to any cone and once again return to center. The object for the rabbit is to run as quickly as possible through a series of cones in any order and sequence that the rabbit desires. The object for the mirroring athlete is to process information and react to the rabbit's movements to mimic the exact path of the rabbit.

At first, only allow the athletes to run while in the box. As the athletes become more advanced at the drill, you can add shuffles, backpedals, and any combination to make the mirroring process more difficult. As with all of the drills, make sure that the athletes demonstrate quality footwork and movement patterns before introducing new skills.

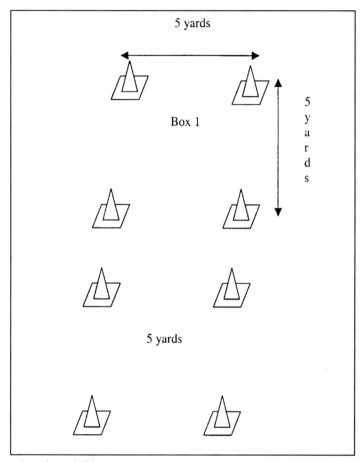

Mirror box drill layout

Shuffling Drill

The open course shuffling drill can be introduced through the use of the shuffle ladder. Through the use of the shuffle ladder, visual and audio cueing can be introduced when the athlete shows proficiency with all shuffling techniques. Balance and fluid transition through each direction change is the goal with shuffle technique. Make sure that the athlete can react and maintain good body mechanics and footwork before introducing mirroring drills.

The shuffle mirroring drill is performed in the same manner as the previously mentioned mirror drills. One athlete will have control of direction changes and the other athlete must attempt to make corresponding changes in direction as quickly as possible. The athlete who is in control can make as many changes as desired. Alternate responsibilities so that each athlete has an opportunity to perform each role. Each working set should have five or more changes in direction.

Chase Drills

Five-Points Drill

The five-points drill is set up in the same manner as the cone drill. In chase drills, one athlete begins at one of the perimeter cones and runs to the center cone, then makes a direction change to any other perimeter cone. From this position, the athlete may proceed to any of the other cones in the course. A second athlete follows the first athlete as soon as he reaches the center cone, and proceeds to follow the first athlete throughout the course. The first athlete's goal is to run through a given number of cones as quickly as possible in any order. The second athlete must attempt to catch up to the first athlete.

Coaching Points:

- The five-points course can be of any desired size. The bigger the course, the easier it will be for the second athlete to follow. The smaller the course, the harder it will be for the second athlete to follow. Keep in mind that the course needs to have enough space for both athletes to move around without running into each other.

- When the athletes can demonstrate quality responsiveness in the drill, allow the athletes to incorporate shuffles, backpedals, and any other footwork combinations.

- Make sure that body positioning is still stressed and quality footwork is focused on. The athletes should continue to lower the hips on deceleration and acceleration phases.

Ball Drops

Ball drops are a great way to develop acceleration. Tennis balls, lacrosse balls, crazy balls, and/or any other ball that will bounce off the surface that is being used will work for these drills. The goal of these drills is to have the athlete begin from a stationary point and gain possession of the ball as quickly as possible.

The drill begins with a coach standing at any given distance from the athlete. The coach then drops or throws the ball(s) in any direction. The athlete must accelerate to the ball as quickly as possible before the ball bounces two times. The coach can keep score or create a competitive twist to the drill by dropping one ball and having two athletes attempt to catch it. This alteration to the drill will not only make the athlete accelerate quickly, but will also teach body positioning and add a competitive nature to the drill.

Ball drops can also be performed with the use of crazy balls, or balls that are not completely round and have protrusions that cause the ball to bounce sporadically when dropped. These balls will add an additional reactive element to ball drills. These drills can also be performed with the athletes beginning on their knees or lying down. The coach may also add an audio component by having the athletes begin with their eyes closed and then starting the drill with a whistle or verbal command to start the drill.

Audio and Visual Cueing Drills

The use of audio and visual cueing should be initiated through the cone drills in this book. Any drill that has multiple direction changes or footwork components can be altered to be an open-style drill. The diamond drill, T-test, rainbow, shuffle ladder, and reaction cuts can all be performed like an open course drill. When the athlete is able to perform drills with audio and visual cues using quality body mechanics and footwork, the athlete can be progressed to cueing drills that are performed without the use of any cones.

The truly open visual and audio cueing drills are performed by having athletes begin from a stationary position and follow cues from the coach. Typically, visual cueing will be easier for the athlete to follow. Multi-directional hand signaling may be the easiest form. Begin with running only for all direction changes and progress to lateral shuffling, backpedals, and even jumps. Again, it is crucial to note that mechanics are the key. Make sure that the athletes are not progressed too quickly. If the athlete cannot maintain mechanics, do not continue with open course drills. Athletes will not benefit from open drills if they cannot perform them correctly.

References and Recommended Reading

1. Abernethy, B. *Acquisition of motor sports*. In F.S. Pyke (Ed.), Better Coaching (pp. 69-98) Canberra, Australian Coaching Council 1991

2. Alricsson, M., Harms-Ringdahl K., Werner S. *Reliability of sports related functional tests with emphasis on speed and agility in young athletes*. Scand J Med Sci Sports. 2001 Aug; 11 (4): 229-32

3. Baechle, T. Earle, R. *Essentials of Strength and Conditioning*. (2nd ed.) Champaign, IL. Human Kinetics, 2002

4. Bompa, T. *Total Training for Young Champions*. Champaign, IL. Human Kinetics, 2000

5. Bompa T. *New Dimensions Regarding Power Training for Sports*. NSCA national convention, Kansas City 1999

6. Brown, L.E., Ferrigno, V.A., Santana, J.C. *Training for Speed, Agility and Quickness*. Champaign, IL; Human Kinetics, 2000

7. Brown T.D. et al *Efficient Arms for Efficient Agility*. Strength and Conditioning Journal. 25. (4) 7-11 2003

8. Burk D. *Year-Round Program Design for Canyon High School Football Players*. NSCA Journal. 17(1) 13-15, 1995

9. Christina, R.W. *Major determinants of the transfer of training: Implications for enhancing sport performance*. In K-W. Kim (Ed), Human performance determinants in sport. (pp.25-52) Seoul, Korea: Korean Society of Sport Psychology. 1996

10. Clark M., Myrland S., Santana J.C., Gambetta V. *Balance, Reaction, Agility, Acceleration, Deceleration: A Comprehensive Approach to Enhancing Human Performance*. NSCA national convention Spokane Wa, 2001

11. Dean, W.P. et al *Efficacy of a 4-week supervised training program in improving components of athletic performance*. Journal of Strength and Conditioning Research 12, 238-242, 1998

12. Grasso, B. *The Concepts of Multilateral Development*, Developing Athletics, On-line Journal, 2003

13. Duvall M. *Implementing Plyometrics in an In-Season Football Program*. NSCA Journal. 15(3): 57-59, 1993

14. Ebben W. *A Review of Football Fitness Testing and Evaluation*. National Strength Conditioning. Assoc. J. 20(1): 42-47, 1998

15. Faccioni A. *Speed Training for Team Sport Athletes*. Faccioni web site, On-line Journal, 2003

16. Faccioni, A. *Principle of Multi-Lateral Development*. Sports Development: Canberra Institute of Technology Lecture 5

17. Faigenbaum, A. *Preseason Conditioning for High School Athletes*. NSCA Journal 23(1) 70-72, 2001

18. Fields, K. Cook, G. *Considering All Angles. Coaching Management* 6.1 Baseball Preseason

19. Foran, B. *High-Performance Sports Conditioning*. Champaign, IL, Human Kinetics, 2001

20. Gambetta, V. *The Daily Special*. Training & Conditioning, 11.8, November 2001

21. Gambetta, V. *Quick to the Ball*. Training & Conditioning, 7.6, December 1997

22. Gambetta, V. *Get Ready, Get Set*. Training & Conditioning, 9.2, March 1999

23. Gambetta, V. *Getting Gait Right*. Training & Conditioning, 11.4, May/June 2001

24. Gambetta V. *The Complete Athlete*. Training & Conditioning, 11.2, March 2001

25. Gambetta V., Gray G. *Following the Functional Path*. Training & Conditioning, 5.2 1995

26. Gambetta V. *Raising the Speed Limit*. Coaching Management 8.7, October 2000

27. Hebert,EP et. Al. *Practice schedule effects on the performance and learning of low-and high-skilled students: an applied study*. Research Quarterly in Exercise and Sport. March; 67 (1):52-8 1996

28. Hellebrandt, F.A. *Physiology of Motor Learning*. Reading in Motor Learning (pp.397-409) Philadelphia, PA; Lea & Febiger

29. Katz J. *NFL Success: Making it to the NFL requires scoring high at the combines. Here's an in-depth look at how to train for the 5-10-5 drill*. Training & Conditioning 7.2, April 1998

30. Kenyon S. *A Conditioning Model For High School Football*. NSCA Journal 16(3) 59-63, 1994

31. LaRosa D. *Year-Round Strength and Conditioning Program for High School Football* NSCA Journal. 17 (1) 7-12, 1995

32. Martinez D. *Is Strength and Conditioning Necessary for the Youth Football Athlete?* NSCA Journal 19(4) 13-17, 1997

33. McHenry, P. *Designing a Plyometric, Speed & Agility Program for High Schools*. York Barbell Magazine, Winter 2000

34. McHenry, P. *Designing a Summer Power/Agility/Speed Program for High School Football*, NSCA Sport Specific Conference, New Orleans 2003

35. Mediate P. *Beyond Strength and Conditioning: Greenwich High School*. NSCA national convention, Kansas City 1999

36. NSCA Coaches College. *Plyometrics & Speed Development*. Colorado Springs, CO. July 9-11, 1999

37. Quan D., et al *The Research on developmental-law of motor coordination ability of children in 7-12 years*. Xi'an Institute of Physical Education, China

38. Palmieri J. *Speed Training for Football*. NSCA Journal 15(6) 12-17, 1993

39. Phelps S. *Teaching Progression*. Speed Quest Newsletter March 2003

40. Phelps S. *Principles, NOT Drills*. Speed Quest Newsletter

41. Plisk S. S. *Agility: Putting Theory into Practice*. NSCA national convention Spokane Wa, 2001

42. Plisk S. S., *The Angle on Agility*. Training & Conditioning, 10.6, September 2000

43. Plisk S. S., Gambetta V. *Tactical Metabolic Training: Part 1*. NSCA Journal 19(2) 44-53, 1997

44. Renfro, G. *Football Power/Agility Drills*. NSCA Journal 19(6) 28-30, 1997

45. Radcliffe, J. *Getting Into Position*. Training and Conditioning 9.3 April 1999

46. Scott, J. *Critical periods in behavioral development*. Science 138 (949-958) 1962

47. Sigmon, C. *The Power of Agility*. Training & Conditioning, 11.4, May/June 2001

48. Smythe, R. *Acts of Agility*. Training & Conditioning, 5.4, August 1995

49. Smythe, R. *Mobility + Ability = Agility*. Coaching Management 4.1 Basketball Preseason 1996

50. Symthe R. *Football SAQ-Speed, Agility, Quickness*. American Football Quarterly

51. Symthe R. *Learning the Quick Step*. Training & Conditioning 6.3, June 1996

52. Young, W.B., Behm, D. *Should Static Stretching Be Used During a Warm-up for Strength and Power Activities*. Strength and Conditioning Journal 12: 33, 2002

53. Young, B. et Al. *Specificity of sprint and agility training methods*. Journal of Strength and Conditioning Research, 15 (3): 315-9 2001

54. Wroblewski G. *Training Camp and In-Season Strength and Conditioning for Football*. NSCA Journal 21(5) 59-64, 1999

About the Authors

Patrick McHenry MA, CSCS*D, PES is the head strength and conditioning coach at Ponderosa High School in Parker, CO. He has a masters in physical education with an emphasis in kinesiology. He is a Certified Strength and Conditioning Specialist with Distinction (CSCS*D), Certified Club Coach with the United States Weightlifting Federation, and a Performance Enhancement Specialist (PES) with the National Academy of Sports Medicine. Patrick has 16 years teaching/coaching experience working with youth, high school, college, and Olympic-level athletes in a wide variety of sports. Patrick has been published in journals, videos, and books. He has also presented at the local, state, and national levels in both strength and conditioning and physical education.

Joel Raether has been an assistant strength and conditioning coach with the University of Denver since the fall of 2002. His primary responsibilities are with men's and women's basketball, men's lacrosse, and skiing. He also assists with the nationally-ranked men's hockey team. Prior to joining the University of Denver strength and conditioning staff, Raether was an assistant strength and conditioning coach at the University of Nebraska at Kearney (2000-2002), where he was responsible for the planning, designing, and administering of strength and conditioning programs for the wrestling, tennis, and track and field teams. He also assisted with training programs for baseball, football, and swimming and helped numerous athletes excel in their respective sport. Raether earned a bachelor of science in exercise science from Nebraska-Kearney in 1999 and continued there through his graduate education, earning a masters of arts and education in exercise science in 2002. Before joining the staff at Nebraska-Kearney, Raether worked as a physical therapy technician with Excel Physical Therapy in Omaha and as a supplemental and dietary research intern with the Exercise Physiology Lab at Kearney, where he published articles related to supplemental and dietary research, as well as sport training articles.